I0425584

Acknowledgements

I wish to express my deep and lasting appreciation to my Father and Mother who cared for me though all those challenging years, and the ongoing love and support my beautiful Mother still gives. To my amazing husband and soul mate Rick Martin for his support and patience as he persistently challenged me to find the answers that would lead to my positive transformation. To my fabulous editor Stew Carter who was supportive and opened my eyes to so many things. To Dr Natasha Turner for her book, The Hormone Diet, that pointed me in the right direction to seek answers. I will also be forever grateful to all the doctors and nurses that helped me though this whole process. Thank you to all the authors of the many books and the NCBI public domain web sites that have served me well in my learning process. And last but not least a very loving, special thank you to my son Richie Martin who has changed my life forever. Because of him I have become who I am today. Thank you, thank you, thank you, I'm very grateful to each and every one of you.

Cindy Martin

INDEX

CHAPTER # 1
In The Beginning

In this chapter I want to share with you some of the challenges and emotions my family and I went through before finding out that I had Celiac Disease. Up until my fortieth Birthday I had more than my share of bloating, diarrhea, cramps, gas, and many trips to doctors and specialists. It was just part of my life until a couple of years ago. But by understanding how I was able to overcome my past misfortunes, misdiagnoses, and disbelief by the medical community imagine how quickly you will be able to change your life without having to experience all the trials and tribulations that I endured on my transformative journey.

It all began when I was a baby. My mother told me that I spent most of my waking hours crying. The doctors told my parents that I had colic, which meant that I cried uncontrollably due to abdominal pain in an otherwise healthy baby. Just a little gas the doctors said - but she should outgrow it by the time she is five months old. But I didn't outgrow it and that is when the doctors started prescribing medication for my mother to give me. I stopped crying, but I was now like a little zombie. So, she decided to take me off the medication and accept the crying over the zombie because there were still those great moments when I was quiet, happy and joyful. I'm grateful that my parents took me off the drug because no one knows what kind of side effects I might have experienced. Mainly because at that time doctors did not explain the side effects of drugs as well as they do now.

So, time went on with the hopes that some day I would outgrow it. As I got older, and the time came that I could talk and express how I was feeling, my parents realized that what they had expected all along was correct. Something wasn't right and it wasn't as simple as just a little gas. But my parents were still puzzled as to what could be wrong with their little girl.

I was given the nickname plain Jane, and you can probably guess why. I didn't like a lot of food and was a very picky eater. I ate my spaghetti as plain noodles, didn't like sodas, and vegetables were totally out of the question. My parents had to wait forever at McDonald's for a hamburger with nothing on it. I can safely say there were more foods I disliked then I liked. But if it contained gluten you could most likely add it to my list of favourite foods. It's sometimes funny how life works - even though it was the very stuff that was making my tummy ache it was my comfort food - and probably is yours as well.

When I began school, this started a whole new set of problems and not just for me, but for my parents as well. It seemed that I needed to take a trip down to the nurse's office everyday just after school started. The school would call mom and she would pick me up. My mom was very stressed, especially because she had just returned to work full time. After this had happened one to many times the school started asking questions of my younger brother such as: "Are we being fed breakfast?" or "Is everything OK at home?". The school started making my mom feel like she wasn't a good parent.

They expressed to her that they felt she was letting a 5-year old manipulate her and if she didn't address the problem it was only going to get bigger. They said I was having an attachment problem and just wanted to stay at home with my mommy. I'm sure I did want to be home with my mommy - who doesn't when they feel sick? My mom was torn as to how she felt. Not knowing whether the school could possibly be right or if her little girl really was sick.

Those of us who are parents can understand the frustration she was experiencing, and because children can be quite clever when it comes to getting their own way, she was beginning to doubt herself. When these medical tests didn't work the school now suspected that there was something else wrong with me. They thought maybe I had a vision problem, or couldn't hear properly, or perhaps had a learning disability. Now along with the long list of different tests that the doctors were doing, I was being subjected to all kinds of different tests at school. I am very grateful that the school worked so hard to try and find out what was wrong. Remember that 40 years ago celiac disease was seldom heard of by doctors, let alone anyone not versed in medicine. Most of all I am thankful that I had a mother and father who were concerned enough to keep fighting to find answers that would relieve the constant pain in my stomach, because it appears they went through a challenging time trying to convince the doctors and the school that there really was something wrong.

My Mom has told me how irritated she felt when this was all happening. But now she is thankful that I was diagnosed with celiac disease, but also saddened to think that all those years of suffering could have been avoided if they had only known. She also confided to me that if she had known that breast feeding me might have given me the antibodies needed to help fight celiac disease, she would have breastfed me. But at that time doctors and hospitals were pushing new mothers to use formula and she thought it would be the right thing to do. Like any new mom she put her faith in the doctors and nurses.

In fairness to doctors and nurses, they are continuously trying to do better and who would have suspected that giving your baby formula, touted as a great advance in pediatrics, rather then breast feeding them could potentially cause the onset of celiac disease or other problems. The research is still not conclusive and continues to this day. Just like some people suspect that genetically modifying wheat may be part of the problems we are faced with now. I guess we should all consider the consequences first and patiently test all new products and procedures for longer time periods to ensure their safety and efficacy, rather then mess with mother nature indiscriminately.

After years of tests and being told that there was nothing wrong with me, I had to accept the predicament I was in. My mind started to build up a tolerance to the pain that the gluten was causing. I began to believe that this was the way a normal body was supposed to feel. One important thing to remember is that even though you have accepted it and are dealing with it in whatever way you can, the damage is still mounting in your body day after day and year after year.

When I finally hit my teen years, I seemed to develop more complications. In hindsight it doesn't surprise me that considering all the stresses of being a teenager - wanting to fit in, be loved, look good, have self worth and numerous other things - that depression set in for years to come. I remember always feeling like I was overweight, and I even went though a stage of being bulimic. I'm a little embarrassed to share this personal experience, but caring about my weight meant that much to me in my teens and I'm sure I was not alone in that. Looking back, I see now that I was far from being overweight. But when you are experiencing inflammation and bloating that makes you look like you're four months pregnant I can understand why I felt I was overweight.

As you can see, I didn't handle stress well or have a good self image. So, with a combination of depression, anxiety, and most of the symptoms of my undiagnosed celiac disease already stressing me along came a new, troubling symptom of vomiting blood which now lead to a new round of testing. My mom would bring me to the hospital when there was blood in my vomit. The doctors would give me a Gravol shot and run more tests. Eventually they came to the conclusion that I had overactive nerves in my stomach. The doctors were of the opinion that the cause was probably stress. This all made perfect sense because most of the other symptoms I was experiencing could be caused by stress as well.

As much as someone doesn't want to be told that they have a problem with stress, especially as a teenager, this was better than nothing. So, I spent a couple more years doing my best to cope with the circumstances. But deep down I knew something wasn't right.

When I turned 19 and moved out with my future husband, Rick, it started to get worse. Which made sense considering my new life style. Of course, being out in the big wide world for the first time with a very limited supply of money and knowledge meant a very poor diet. There were a lot of breads, noodles, baked treats and processed foods; things that fill a belly quickly, and not an abundance of foods that were good for me, let alone gluten free. Looking back, I know that a lot of the foods that were cheap, fast, easy to cook and tasted so good had gluten in them, after all gluten is used as a filler. I also started drinking beer, which I realized I couldn't handle very well since I usually vomited, passed out or fainted and would occasionally have small seizures.

Of course, I didn't want to listen to Rick nagging me about going to get tested. He kept saying that there had to be something wrong, and God only knows how much I didn't want to have any more doctors hypothesize about what else may potentially be wrong. So, the bathroom became a good place for me to deal with my new problems and there I could hide them from everybody. I knew it was bad; bouncing my head off the toilet as I fell and cleaning up vomit off the floor.

But soon I learned how to keep myself safe. I found if I lay down on the floor when I first started to feel this way or went right to bed that it would all be okay (or so I thought) and I could control the end results better and still keep everyone from finding out. Looking back, I can't believe I did this because having seizures or fainting should not to be taken lightly. The seizures and fainting continued until I stopped drinking completely. It reached the point that I couldn't even get though one drink. Keep in mind that any alcohol made with gluten is not safe. It probably won't affect you the way it affected me, but it still contains gluten and that will damage your intestines. I have put together a list of things that contain gluten and chapter 6 contains that list.

So, for the next ten years I had to manage life with all my issues, and I just kept most of it to myself. I am sure my husband Rick saw it a little differently, he would say that I was sick a lot and that I was complaining most of the time. It is funny how we can sometimes see the same events so differently when one is looking from the inside out and the other is looking from the outside in.

When I was pregnant with my son, I developed a life-threatening complication called H.E.L.L.P syndrome. H.E.L.L.P. stands for: H: Hemolysis which is the rupturing of red blood cells; EL: Elevated Liver enzymes; and LP: low platelet count. This is said to be a variant or complication to pre-eclampsia but could also occur for unknown reasons. Women with autoimmune conditions may have a higher chance of HELLP or pre-eclampsia. This explained a lot for me since I always felt that there might have been a link once I had found out I had celiac disease, which is also an autoimmune disease. If you

[8]

would like to read more about my pregnancy and my little miracle, I have written about it at the end of the book in chapter 10.

The Later Years

After years of my husband nagging me to seek help, I finally went for another colonoscopy and blood work (but not for celiac disease). I was told I had Irritated Bowel Syndrome (IBS), the precise cause of which is not known. Now I had a new diagnosis and I began researching this diagnosis so I could start taking steps to help myself. In spite of that things were still not improving and I was losing my faith in the ability of the doctors to diagnose my problems.

Just before my 40th birthday my husband was listening to a talk radio show and the topic was a book called The Hormone Diet by Dr. Natasha Turner. As he listened, he realized that this could be my problem. When he arrived home that night, he was excited to share all the interesting things he learned from the talk show and suggested I get the book. I was excited at the prospect of finding something that might hold the answers to my problems.

It was a beautiful May weekend and some friends of ours had taken us out for dinner and a show. We were celebrating my birthday and theirs as well. Between dinner and the show Rick asked me if I would like to go and get the book, he was so excited about, The Hormone Diet, and of course I jumped at the idea. We left immediately and ran to the book store to see if we could find the book he had talked about. Of course, the book was there because fate had determined that I was supposed to read it so I could get one step closer to solving my puzzle. This turned out to be a birthday present from him that I would never forget because it was bringing me closer to resolving my problems.

When I started reading this book I thought, "Wow, this could be it". Even though it wasn't completely what my problem was, there was some amazing information that pointed me in the right direction to soon find the truth. So, I thank you, Dr. Natasha Turner, for opening my eyes to possibilities I had never thought of. It was her book that recommended starting with an anti-inflammatory detoxification. That made me now realize that I had a serious inflammation problem, and it looked like this stuff called gluten was the biggest part of my problem. So, I tried to stop eating this stuff called gluten, that I was just finding out about.

It was hard, gluten was everywhere and it's not like there was an area in the grocery store in 2009 that was allotted to gluten free foods. I had good days, but was still having a lot of bad days, but those good days kept me going and trying to find out more.

I continued on my journey to try and find things to eat like breads and all the other goodies that didn't have gluten, but this was not turning out well. All I could find was vacuum packed bread full of many chemicals I couldn't even pronounce, as well as due dates that were months away. I found if I stayed on just fruits and vegetables my body was delighted but my spirits were not high. I remember being very discouraged and hating my predicament. I just didn't understand any of it. How could food make you sick and especially the foods I loved and had been eating all my life.

My mom was also having problems with her stomach around this time and had decided to go for a blood test for food intolerance testing. After seeing how this made so many things better for her, I wanted to see if it could help me. I had still not completely fixed my problems, and I may have been dragging my feet a bit. My husband decided to give me the money to get this blood test done as a gift for Valentines day (this gift was better than chocolate). The cost was $500 which was a lot of money for a test that I thought should be freely offered as a medical test. The test results came back and there it was - a intolerance to wheat and 40 other items.

By now it was time for one of my routine colonoscopies. The nurse that was getting me ready for the procedure suggested that I ask the doctor for an endoscopy procedure as well. I'm very grateful to her for that suggestion. It also helped that I had the results of the food intolerance test. So now I knew that I had celiac disease because the doctor confirmed that damage had taken place to the villi in my intestines. Even though I had taken some steps by trying to eat gluten-free this was the big push I needed to take full control of my life. Now it was time to take the rest of the steps and become completely gluten free for the rest of my life.

CHAPTER 2

What Is Celiac Disease And How Does It Differ From A Wheat Allergy And Gluten Sensitivity?

Celiac (also spelled coeliac) disease is a genetic autoimmune disorder that can affect children and adults. This disease makes the body unable to digest or absorb certain proteins, called gluten, found in wheat, rye, and barley, which are commonly used to produce foods such as breads, pasta, cookies, cakes, prepackaged foods and many other products that will be listed in chapter 6. When gluten is consumed the body's immune system responds, and causes damage to the villi (tiny finger like projection) in the small intestines.

The villi can become completely flattened from years of damage. Damage to the villi causes the body to be unable to absorb nutrients into the body from food that is eaten. The only way to repair the villi is to go on a completely gluten free diet and remain on it for the rest of your life.

Celiac disease is *not* the same as a wheat allergy or gluten sensitivity. A brief summary of the differences is explained below.

A wheat allergy causes the body to generate allergy-causing antibodies (allergens) to proteins found in wheat. Wheat allergies can have some of the same symptoms as celiac disease but may also cause hives, skin rash, stuffy or runny nose, sneezing and Anaphylaxis (less common), a life-threatening reaction that impairs breathing and sends the body into shock.

If you have gluten sensitivity you will still be affected by wheat, rye, barley and anything else containing gluten. You may even experience some of the same symptoms as a person suffering from celiac disease. But the big difference is that your small intestines won't be permanently damaged by eating gluten and you may outgrow the intolerance.

So, as you can see all three have the same source, wheat (or the gluten it contains), but generate different reactions in different people. The four reactions can range from none in a healthy person who is unaffected by wheat or gluten, to an immediately life-threatening reaction in people who suffer from wheat allergy and anything in between including the life-long debilitating effects of celiac disease.

What is Gluten

Gluten Is the generic name for some of the proteins (shown by % of proteins in the grain that are gluten) found in wheat (approximately 69%), barley (46%-52%), rye (30%-50%) and many other grains. Gluten proteins are stretchy and sticky, and act like a glue that binds all of our favourite foods like cakes, pastry and breads. It's gives the amazing chewy, spongy texture by allowing doughs to have the big bubbles that make breads and cakes lighter and chewier. It can also be used as a filler, a stabilizer and a thickening agent. In fact, gluten can be purchased in most grocery stores and is added to the flour used in some recipes. It helps boost the flavours in things like soups, ice cream, salad dressings and many other foods. As you can see gluten could potentially be used in many products in small amounts to make them taste better, feel better and have more mouth appeal.

CHAPTER 3

Starting The Journey To Transform Your Life

So now it's time to make some life altering changes that will make you feel healthy, pain free, lighter and happier. You will experience how you are supposed to feel all the time. One of the first things I did to start my transformation was to go on a 'Process of Elimination' diet, and it did not cost anything. By trying this diet first, I was able to find the foods that were causing my problems and find out what foods I could eat without problem. You might try this diet and find out that it is not wheat at all that is causing your problems, but something completely different. I am not going to pretend that this process is easy because it is not. It is going to be emotional - and trying at times, but the end results will blow you away. You won't believe your body is supposed to feel this good- trust me on that. When you are ready to start this diet follow the instructions that are provided in the next couple of pages to get the best results, and it will make a major improvement in your life. You should also consult your medical practitioner to ensure that you can follow this diet, especially if you have health conditions or are under medical care.

PROCESS OF ELIMINATION DIET

Foods To Include

Foods To Exclude

Fruits

Fresh or frozen – almost all types

Citrus fruits – such as oranges, grapefruit, lemon, lime etc.

Vegetables

Almost all vegetables – raw, fresh, steamed or sautéed

Eggplant

Tomatoes

Corn

Peppers

Starches

Rice – all types

Buckwheat

Quinoa

Amaranth

Teff

Tapioca

Wheat

Bran

Corn

Spelt

Oats

Gamut

Rye

Barley

Triticale

Gluten containing products

Legumes

All beans

Lentils

Peas

Tofu

Soybean

Tempeh

Nuts and Seeds

All seeds and nuts

Meats and Fish

Chicken, organic

Turkey, organic

Lamb

Fresh fish

Duck

Wild game

Beef

Pork

Chicken eggs

Shellfish

Canned Meats

Processed meats such as cold cuts, hot dogs and bacon

Dairy and Dairy Substitutes

Unsweetened coconut milk

Rice milk

Milk

Butter

Yoghurt

Cream cheese

Cottage cheese

Real cream

(no dairy products of any form)

Fats

Cold pressed olive oil

Olive oil

Coconut oil

Flax seed oil

Any hydrogenated oil

Margarine

Salad dressing

Processed oil

Mayonnaise

Spices and Condiments

Pepper

Ketchup

Sea salt	Mustard
Himalayan pink salt	Relish
Ginger	Soy sauce
Oregano	Vinegar
Dill	Barbecue sauce
Rosemary	Any spice not listed in the Foods to Include column
Parsley	
Turmeric	
Cumin	

Sweeteners

Stevia	White sugar
	Brown sugar
	Maple syrup
	Corn syrup
	Fructose
	Honey

For about 3 to 4 weeks avoid all foods listed above in the right column. This will give your body time to detoxify (detox). Drink water, lots of it - 2.5 litres (10 cups) for women and 3.5 litres (14 cups) for men every day. This will help in the process of flushing toxins out of the body. If this diet is used for children not as much water is required and the time should be reduced to 2 to 3 weeks. Only 1.5 to 2 litres (6 to 8 cups) for between 8 and 12 years old and 1 litre (4 cups) for children who are 5 to 8 years old. Children under 5 years old should not be following this regimen without medical supervision. Keep in mind that this includes all fluid intake (for a detox fluid intake should be just water for best results). If you have any existing allergies continue to keep them out of this process

Reintroduction

When you have completed the 3 to 4 weeks (2 to 3 for children) you should be feeling very different. More energetic, no bloating and maybe even a bit lighter. Because this will reduce the physical pain you should start feeling happier. I always knew when I was experiencing inflammation (bloating) in my body because my rings wouldn't slip on and off my finger easily. If you are still feeling bloated and are having problems, then it may be something else that is bothering you. It's possible it could be one or more of the spices or other foods on the good list. The more you remove the more likely you are to discover what foods you are intolerant to. You already have a lot of time invested in this so keep going. We are all different so it is hard to pinpoint the exact intruder(s) that may be causing the problems. If you have tried all the things listed above and you are still not feeling relief, I suggest you seek medical attention.

Most of you will be feeling this magical new body and will want to start the reintroduction of foods, slowly and one at a time, so you can monitor yourself for symptoms. Choose a food group and reintroduce one food at a time. I would recommend starting with vegetables and then fruit, there is less chance of them being the problem. For example, on Monday allow a vegetable back into your diet, maybe tomatoes, but just for that day. Then monitor your body for the next two days. On day four try another vegetable and repeat the process. Do not add too many vegetables all at once.

Keep a journal to record things like bowel movements - how many, loose or solid etc., gastrointestinal (GI) pain, skin breakouts, joint pain, inflammation, mood swings and types, energy, sleep patterns, headaches and bloating. If there is any thing else that you notice or that feels different than how you were feeling after the detox make sure you write it down. Keeping the journal will help you to track all the things that you experience. This whole process will take approximately 6 to 10 weeks. Just remember that at the end of all the hard work, it will be well worth it. Also try and remember not to add too many things back in at once. This way you can pin point the foods that are causing you problems. If you pay close attention your body will be telling you exactly what foods are causing you the problems. So, listen closely to what it is telling you and record it all in the journal.

This process of elimination diet worked for me at first, but it wasn't enough to keep me off the foods that caused me problems. I needed to have something in writing because after all the years that I had felt betrayed by this body I doubted my ability to trust it. Because this is something, I have struggled with most of my life it had always caused me to have low self worth.

When I was diagnosed with Ulcerative Colitis, I had to follow a very strict diet that would help heal my body and get my flair up under control, it was an elimination diet. This diet had to be low fiber and easily digestible. I was down to 25 foods items, everything had to be peeled, cooked and pureed and I didn't reintroduction anything for 3 weeks. This was a very successful diet and I was able to get my flair up under control. I guess being diagnosed with this disease was enough to make me stay away from the foods that were the problems. For more information on Ulcerative colitis see chapter 8.

Here is a list of the top 8 food people are allergic too – milk (dairy), peanut, tree nuts (almonds, cashews, walnuts) fish, shellfish, eggs, soya, wheat, and I would add corn as well. I would wait as long as possible to reintroduce these foods.

CHAPTER 4

Getting Tested

By now you probably have a pretty good idea of what foods are causing you difficulty. If you found that you experienced most of your problems when you reintroduced things like wheat, barley, rye, or anything else containing gluten it is a good indication that you probably have gluten intolerance, celiac disease or wheat allergy. Your body should know best but it is always a good idea to be tested to have it confirmed.

First you will want to book an appointment to see your family doctor. Whether you have done a 'Process of Elimination' diet (refer to Chapter 3) or not, you will want to express your thoughts and concerns. If you have followed the diet and kept a journal, as recommended, while you were reintroducing the food groups this can be presented to the doctor to assist in the diagnosis. But even if you don't have a food list you can still share the symptoms you are experiencing.

It's a good idea to make a list of the questions and things you would like to say to the doctor because if you're like me you won't remember most of the things you wanted to discuss and before you know it your appointment is finished and nothing has been resolved. It wasn't until I started writing everything down before I went to see my doctor, and taking that list with me, that I felt confident that I was getting my point across. So, don't be like me and experience years of suffering when you can take control of your health right now. Just **MAKE A LIST** and take it with you. I have written down some examples of things that should be on the list so you can have an idea of how to start your list and what should be on it. This list is not exhaustive and is intended to be a guideline. Your list should be about you and your symptoms, you may have more, or less, or different ones, but these are some of the ones commonly associated with negative reactions to gluten and wheat.

Things You Should Share With Your Doctor

Express your symptoms: Do you have bloating, diarrhea, constipation, cramping, fatigue, weight gain or loss, depression, hives, nausea, indigestion, gas pain or any other symptoms?

How often: Which of the symptoms you are experiencing are continuous and which are occasional?

When: When did these symptoms start? Have they become worse?

Share: Share with your doctor any other conditions you may have that may be related to celiac disease - like another autoimmune diseases, anemia, and any of the other conditions that I have listed later in this book in Chapters 7 and 8.

Prescriptions and Vitamins: Ensure your doctor is aware of any vitamins or prescriptions you might be taking.

Journal: Ensure you share your journal from the Process of Elimination diet if you have one. Share with the doctor foods that you found affected you, and tell him or her what you experience when you eat them or eliminate them (remember that if you have gone completely gluten free it may affect most of the test results). This is because there will be no antibodies in your blood - which I explain more about under the blood testing section.

Things You Can Ask Your Doctor

As well as sharing with the doctor everything you have been experiencing you might have some questions for him or her such as:

What are the different types of tests that will determine if I have celiac disease, wheat allergy or wheat intolerance?

If I have celiac disease will you check for vitamin or mineral deficiencies?

And ask anything else you would like to know more about.

The more information and opinions you have the better it will be on your journey to better health. Now that you have taken the first step with your visit to the doctor, hopefully he or she will be setting up appointments for some tests or to see a specialist who will be conducting the tests.

Here Are Some of The Different Types of Tests

Blood Test

Tissue Transglutaminase Antibodies test (tTG) IgG is a test that is carried out on blood that is drawn from your arm. The lab technicians look for antibodies in the blood. The body produces antibodies in the blood to fight off any intruder. In this case they are looking for the antibodies that the body produces when it is reacting to **GLUTEN**. This test is also effective in evaluating whether you are still eating foods contaminated by gluten after you are on your gluten free diet.

Genetic Testing

Genetic testing can be performed on a sample of blood, skin, or hair. People with celiac disease carry one or both marker genes. The marker genes they are looking for are HLA-DQ2 and HLA-DQ8. Just because you are a carrier of these marker genes it does not mean you will ever develop celiac disease.

Colonoscopy Test

A Colonoscopy Test (formerly called a colonostrophy) is a procedure used by a doctor or a trained specialist who inserts a long, flexible, narrow tube with a tiny camera and a light on the end of it into the colon. This tool is called an endoscope, but medical terminology calls the tool by the organ that it is being used to examine because it has been specifically adapted for that purpose (see image following). He or she will insert the tube into your anus to look inside the rectum, colon, large intestine and at the base of your small intestine. Before you are scheduled for the procedure you will be given instructions to follow at home to prepare yourself. You will have to perform a bowel preparation. This process is used to clean out your large intestines (colon). This will cause diarrhea so you may want to stay close to a bathroom. As well, you will have to strictly follow a clear liquid diet for 1 to 3 days before and avoid drinks that have red or purple dyes. On the day of the procedure at the hospital or outpatient centre a health care professional (nurse) will place an intravenous (IV) needle in your arm to give you a sedative, anaesthetic and/or pain medication so you can relax during the procedure. Because of this you will have to arrange a ride home. You will have to stay a couple of hours until the sedative wears off. You will be on your side on a table while the above procedure is being performed. There will be a nurse checking your vital signs and keeping you comfortable. The camera on the end of the long flexible tube will send video back to a monitor so they can examine the colon in real time during the procedure. You may not remember any of the procedure, or you may remember some or all of it, depending on the strength of the anaesthetic that has been administered. *I always remember being in the room with the doctor and nurses just before the procedure, then I would be out like a light and wake up later in the recovery room with a lot of gas.* Gas is common after the procedure because the intestine is expanded slightly with air for easier viewing - so don't be embarrassed because likely half of the people in your recovery room are there for the same procedure and if not, chances are they have been though this at some time in their lives. As well as the gas, you may have abdominal cramping or bloating for about an hour after the procedure. There are reasons Doctors give you a colonoscopy. It can help them find unexplained symptoms such as:

changes in your bowel activity like diarrhea or constipation;

bleeding from your anus;

pain in your abdomen; and

unexplained weight loss.

Doctors also perform colonoscopies to look for the evidence of colon or rectal cancer, Crohn's disease, colitis, and polyps; and they might be able to see evidence of celiac disease at the base of the small intestine. So, you can probably understand when looking at the reasons they perform colonoscopies, that some of the symptoms are the same as celiac disease. I've had too many colonoscopies over the years and celiac disease was never found; but I understand now that the doctors were doing what they felt they needed to do. So, in my opinion this is not the route to go when looking for celiac disease.

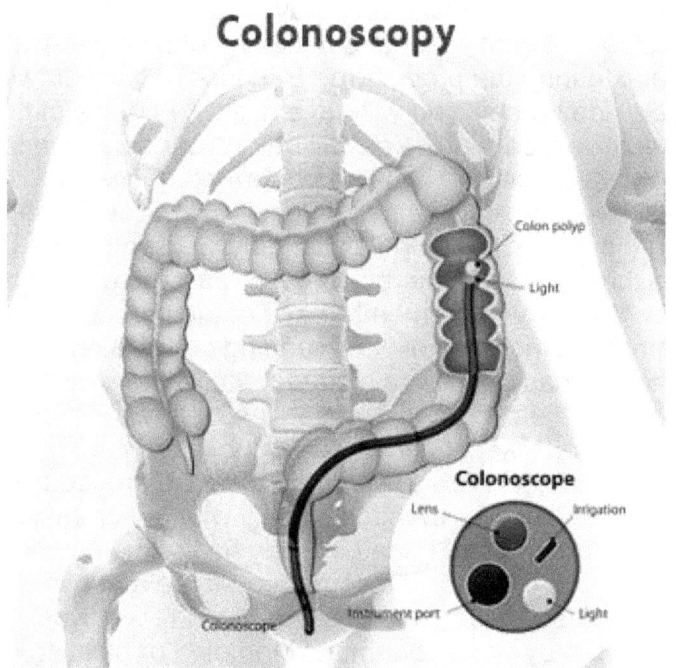

Upper Gastrointestinal (GI) Endoscopy Procedure

Upper GI gastrointestinal endoscopy is a procedure that uses an endoscope to examine the esophagus, stomach and duodenum (first part of small intestine). You will have this procedure performed in a hospital or outpatient centre. Much the same as a colonoscopy, you will have an IV needle placed in your arm. This is how you will be given your sedative to make sure you are comfortable and relaxed for the procedure. Your vital signs will be monitored during the procedure. You will be put on a table on your side. Your doctor will insert the endoscope down your esophagus, into your stomach and into your duodenum. They will pump air into your stomach and small intestine so they can see things better. The camera on the end of the long flexible tube will send a video back to a monitor so they can examine the lining of your upper GI tract. As well they will be doing a full examination for abnormalities and general health. They will take a biopsy of the tissue at this time if required. The reason doctors perform this procedure is to check for conditions such as cancer, celiac disease, Crohn's disease and gastritis. The biopsy is needed to diagnose these conditions. Your doctor will also give you a list of instructions to follow before you come for the procedure, like no food or drink for 8 hours before. And you will have to arrange a ride home because the sedative used during the procedure may not have worn off before you are released. You will also have to stay at the hospital for up to 2 hours after to make sure all is well. You may feel nausea or bloating and you may have a sore throat for up to 2 days after the procedure.

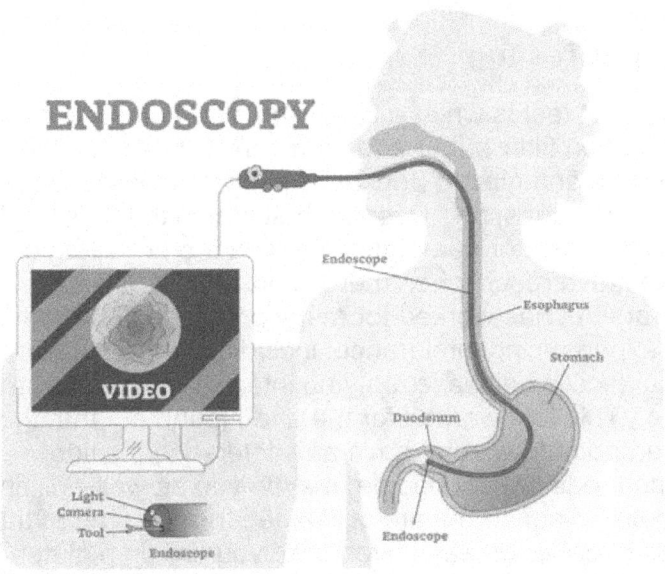

ENDOSCOPY

Stool Testing

Three types of antibodies, anti-gliadin, (IgA, IgG, IgE) will be commonly produced in your body to fight against the gliadin part of gluten, whether it is from an intolerance, allergy or celiac disease. It won't be known which one you have when they measure it in the lab. Stool testing is sometimes done to check for the specific anti-gliadin antibody called IgA. This antibody is produced by the body when it reacts to gliadin. Testing positive will show your doctor that further diagnostic testing for celiac disease is required. The doctor will provide you with a sterile container for collecting the sample. You will receive instructions on how to collect the sample to prevent contamination.

Saliva Testing

This test is performed to analyze a saliva specimen for the same antibodies as mentioned in the stool testing, IgA, but can also find antibody IgG. If they are present then further testing will be required to check for celiac disease.

Dried Blood Spot Testing

A dried blood spot test is when a small sample of blood from your fingertip is put on filter paper and then sent to a lab. At the lab it will be checked for anti-gliadin (IgG and IgA) antibodies which are attacking the foods in question. Despite the chance that this might give you a positive result for something that you are not allergic to it rarely gives a negative result when there is an allergy. This test is not 100% accurate but has worked for many people to find foods to which they are experiencing intolerance, including wheat. It won't tell you if you have celiac disease, only an intestinal biopsy will tell you this for sure. This test worked for me and I found out that there were many other foods to which I have an intolerance, besides gluten containing foods. Many people, maybe you as well, will find that you have celiac disease but are still experiencing some of the same symptoms of celiac disease even after you are on a gluten free diet. This could be because there are other foods bothering you and this test can help you to find some of these and perhaps provide some relief.

Capsule Endoscopy

A Capsule Endoscopy is a miniature video camera that is in the form of an oversized pill that is swallowed. This procedure allows video images of the lining of the gut to be taken on its journey through the intestines. The doctor will be able to view the entire small intestine, not just the top one or two feet. They will be able to view the complete journey until the camera is passed in your stool. It sends information to a recorder which you will wear as a belt. The journey will take about 8 hrs. The only preparation is to not eat or drink anything for about half a day. The one problem with this test is they are not able to take a biopsy. This test could also be done to follow up on patients with celiac disease to make sure they are not still suffering from damage to their intestines.

Brighter Future

The future is looking bright for people who want to know if they have celiac disease. It looks like a new blood test might be available in the near future for people already following a gluten free diet. I am just hearing about it as I write this book and I feel that this could be wonderful news for people who think that they have celiac disease but don't want to start eating gluten again just so the test can be carried out.

As you can see there are many different tests out there that will help you get closer to the truth about what is going on in your body. There should be no reason why you shouldn't be able to have something done if you suspect celiac disease. You are in a great time where doctors are much more aware of celiac disease, wheat intolerance and wheat allergy. Take advantage of it because it was not talked about when I was sick several years ago. But I am grateful that it is recognized now for all people reading this book.

CHAPTER 5

Getting Results

If the results of the tests discussed in Chapter 4 come back and it has the life changing news that you have celiac disease, a wheat allergy or gluten intolerance then that is one step closer to feeling absolutely tremendous. If there is a restriction or limitation on the wheat in your diet there are many other foods to please your palate out there. And in many cases, this is the trigger to expand your diet into some new and unexplored gastronomic areas that will have your mouth watering in anticipation. In the next chapter there is a list of foods you can eat and foods you should avoid.

Now that you know what has been causing all these complications, you are going to have to make some changes in your life. You are going to want to figure out how much you want this to work for you. It's like quitting smoking or giving up alcohol - you may not succeed the first or second time, but the main thing is that you keep working at eliminating gluten from your diet. The longer you go without it, the more you will see how incredible you feel without the pain it causes, and every time you have a set back it will show you how unpleasant it makes you feel. Remember - it's not how many times you get knocked down that is important, it's how many times you get back up that matters.

There have been many studies on animals and humans that have shown how some foods are very addictive. Just like cocaine and heroin some foods can trigger the pleasure centres of the brain. Chemicals like dopamine, serotonin, oxytocin and endorphins, the feel-good hormones are released into the brain. The brain remembers that the foods you ate are what gave you this extraordinary feeling and wants more. Usually it is sugars, salts and fats that generate the addiction, but new studies are finding that refined flours and gluten are causing similar effects.

I know from first hand experience the addiction to gluten - I wanted it all the time. It would take me 2 to 3 weeks to stop craving the breads and pastas. But if I had something that contained gluten the challenge was to conquer and control my emotions, because even though I had a lot of discomfort my brain associated those foods with feeling good and would release the feel-good chemicals making the cycle hard to break. But over time I broke the cycle and created new neural pathways in my brain. These new pathways take time to develop, and that demands a lot of discipline. But you can do it, as I did. Have faith and know in your heart that you can succeed, just like so many others who were able to make adjustments to their behaviour over time.

Once the new neural pathways in your brain are developed it becomes much easier to follow a gluten free diet. But be cautious when you stop eating all the foods that contain gluten because you may want to replace them with other foods that are going to trigger the feel-good hormones. Foods that contain a lot of sugar, starches, salts and fat. Just as when a smoker stops smoking, they sometimes turn to eating more to replace the mouth appeal of the cigarette and the nicotine, these sweet, starchy, salty and fatty foods can often be the replacement sought out when coming off gluten because they will trigger the release of the feel-good chemicals in the brain.

The best thing you can do for yourself is to duct tape your mouth and lock your self in a room. Well we all know we can't live like that so you could try eating an abundance of fruits and vegetables and drink plenty of water, or do a natural food detoxification (detox) as discussed in Chapter 3 (check with your doctor first). This would be the fastest way of getting your body to feel marvellous and healthy. I would recommend a natural food detox without taking anything that flushes out the colon. When the gut is flushed out all bacteria are removed because nothing we do can distinguish between good and bad bacteria. The good bacteria are ones like lactobacillus and Bifidobacterium and millions of others that help with digestion, detoxification and our overall health. Taking a probiotic is recommended after doing a detox.

We need bacteria in our body and more good bacteria in our

[29]

body means less bad bacteria. Good bacteria provide us with the energy and building blocks that our bodies need. They work best on good foods like fruits and vegetables and of course the bad bacteria tend to take the sugars and refined carbohydrates and make them into fats and other bad things such as plaque and cholesterol. Therefore, I don't recommend a colon flush because a colon flush can't distinguish the difference between good and bad bacteria - it just wipes them all out. I made the mistake of taking something that gave me a colon flush and I was very sick for months as my body rebelled against a colon that was wiped clean of all bacteria, both good and bad.

Research is showing us that when they have looked at the gut of someone with celiac disease, they are missing some of the key good bacteria (microbiota). The researchers feel that the microbiota in our gut plays a huge role in preventing disease manifestation as well as weight control problems (obesity). Current research is even indicating that this microbiome is linked to autism. Creating a good microbiome is extremely important for more than the obvious digestive reasons as research links it to more and more diseases, even as far as brain disorders.

CHAPTER 6

Living With Celiac Disease

In this chapter, I will share a list of foods that are gluten free and a list of foods to avoid. I will also share a list of products that may contain gluten, some of which will surprise you. Also, I will explain what to look for on labels when buying foods, as well as clarifying how to avoid cross-contamination.

What does living gluten free mean? It means you will have to increase your awareness. You will have to decipher labels to see where gluten is hidden, and become more mindful of everything you are eating, and as you will see, other places it is hiding such as makeup, vitamins and supplements. You will have to ensure that you are aware of how your food has been prepared. You are also going to have to make some transformations in your home and life outside your home. But most of all you are going to have to improve how you deal with your emotions. Emotions such as *fear* of eating gluten, *distrust* in who and how the food has been prepared, *anger* because you can't eat the foods you crave anymore and, of course, *sadness* that this is happening to you.

When I first found out that I had Celiac Disease I was in a troubled, depressed state and I didn't think it would be possible to live without all the foods that contain gluten. The crazy part was that I didn't have any idea how many items contained gluten. In the beginning I found it extremely hard to avoid gluten. But I soon found out that I had to educate myself on how to read labels, as well as figure out the words that meant gluten was in the food. Once I got familiar with the list of foods to avoid, things got a little easier when I was shopping or eating out. It took several years before I didn't have to take out my list of 'Foods to Avoid' when shopping or the rare times we were eating out.

Eating out was the biggest hurdle. My son played a lot of sports and we couldn't always eat at home. At that time there wasn't a huge selection of places I could eat, whether it was fast food or a restaurant. There are many more fast foods places and restaurants offering gluten free food now. But keep in mind that the chance of cross contamination will always be there if you are not preparing your own food.

Cross Contamination

What is cross contamination? Cross contamination is when food you have eaten has come in contact with gluten during preparation. Examples: When gluten free food is being fried or cooked with food that has gluten on it or in it or the food is prepared on the same counter or cutting board and it hasn't been cleaned. When the person preparing your food doesn't wash their hands before preparing the gluten free food or wears gloves that were used to handle foods containing gluten. Also, gluten free foods stored in the same place as gluten containing foods. There are many restaurants claiming to offer gluten free and because of these claims there have been many individuals investigating these claims on their own, the conclusion being it's not as safe as we would like to think.

Some new tests that are being carried out are finding that even when a food is labelled gluten free it may have traces of gluten. If the grower uses the same machinery for harvesting and/or transporting gluten free grains and grains that contain gluten it is possible that some cross contamination could occur. It may be that the machinery used to process gluten free grains may have been previously used to process gluten containing grains and not properly cleaned.

There are many ways that gluten can accidentally end up on your food so keep in mind that you can never be 100% safe if you eat processed foods. One way to ensure your safety is to only eat fruits and vegetables. Also, ensure that when dining out you express, in a positive polite way, to the wait staff or person preparing the food that you have celiac disease.

I would like to share some of my dining out experiences so that you get a better understanding of what can happen. My husband and I went to a place that made submarine sandwiches and they had gluten free bread. I was excited that I could have a sub until I saw the person prepare my husband's sandwich and then use the same gloves to prepare mine. That was the last time I went to that place. Another time, we went to a restaurant that listed a lot of gluten free foods on their menu. I ordered a plate of french fries and when I got to the bottom of the plate, I noticed something on my plate that looked like a small piece of a chicken nugget – and they have a coating containing flour.

You will have to decide if it is worth the risk to go out for a meal. If you enjoy eating out then you should be mindful of what and where you are eating. Look at everything you are putting in your mouth, you might notice something that doesn't look right and this could mean that it has been in contact with gluten.

Another hurdle I had to overcome was going out for dinner at other peoples' houses. You cannot expect everyone to know what gluten is and accommodate your needs, even if they did invite you. If they are able to accommodate some of your needs, be grateful. Don't be frustrated just because they don't have a gluten free desert. Always remember that it is not their fault that you can't consume gluten and the sooner you get over playing the victim the better your experiences will be. Think of what you have, not what you don't have.

Acceptance is the only way that you can move forward in your positive transformation. Keep in mind that you still may end up with cross contamination, even though family, friends and restaurants are doing their best to accommodate you. They may not know what to look for or how easily cross contamination can occur. You need to express the seriousness of keeping gluten away from you to ensure your safety. You can always explain your needs and ask questions to ensure the chances of consuming gluten are minimized. Ensure you do this in a compassionate, helpful way because firstly they don't want to harm you and have a lawsuit or food safety violation and secondly the restaurants want to keep customers returning so they stay in business.

Here is another example I would like to share with you. It was a very common thing where I worked to have breakfast cooked for us on the weekend. Usually one person would cook for all of us and up to 7 people might be having breakfast together. I had built up some trust in my co worker. He had been cooking breakfast for all of us and was always very careful to cook my food first. I even brought in a toaster from home just for my

[33]

bread. On this particular day only about 15 minutes after I had finished this amazing breakfast that he had generously cooked for all of us I started feeling like I had food poisoning. I was feeling terrible with cramping and dreadful diarrhea. I called my co-worker and asked him if there was any chance that something, we ate for breakfast had gluten in it. He assured me that he was positive it was all safe from the possible contamination that I was suspicious of. Hours later when he was throwing out the garbage, he looked at the sausage pack and realized they contained wheat crumble. I hadn't given the sausages a second thought when I was eating them because they had always been safe before. But he had accidentally grabbed the wrong ones from home when getting ready to come to work - and these ones were not gluten free.

The reason I've shared these stories with you is to show you that even though the people preparing your food have the best intentions and don't want to harm you, it may happen. You must look out for your health - so remember that you are taking a chance any time you don't eat at home or prepare your own food and bring it with you. Something else to keep in mind is to always read the ingredients because manufacturers sometimes change the ingredients in something you have been eating, and although it was safe at one time it may no longer be safe the next.

Something I had to start doing was to pack a lunch for myself. The only problem with this is that it takes some planning. You will have to make sure you have foods at home that you can bring with you. Make sure that the things you are packing are going to be things that you look forward to eating. Such as your favourite nuts, toasted coconut, raisins, dates, gluten free crackers, energy bars, cookies, a sandwich made with gluten free bread, fruits, vegetables and any other thing you might like to bring that will make you feel cheerful and satisfied.

At first, I was miserable, bitter and jealous because I couldn't have the foods I wanted and my husband and son looked like they were enjoying their meals so much. It's not like it was their fault that I couldn't eat those foods any more but I was still jealous. Learning how to master my emotions and what I was thinking was very difficult. I guess I thought that they were supposed to stop eating everything I couldn't eat. I'm probably not the only one who has felt this way but the faster you can

[34]

recognize and control your negative emotions the better you will be in the long run. Try to think about how grateful you are for knowing and being able to control what it is that causes your body so many difficulties.

Reading a label

Back in 2004, in the United States, the Food Allergen Labeling and Consumer Protection Act was signed. Wheat is one of the 8 major foods that are considered the biggest problems for food allergies along with milk, eggs, fish (e.g., bass, flounder, cod), Crustacean shellfish (e.g., crab, lobster, shrimp), tree nuts (e.g., almonds, walnuts, pecans), peanuts and soybeans. These 8 foods have to be listed on the label if the product contains them.

On 5 Aug 2014 the U.S Food and Drug Administration (FDA) passed that if you are going to voluntarily label something "Gluten Free" it must meet the requirements of the agency's gluten free labelling rules. This gluten free labelling states that a product claiming to be gluten free must have less then 20 parts per million (ppm) of gluten in it. You can find out more information at https://www.fda.gov. If you click on this site, then type gluten free labelling laws or food allergy labelling laws into the search bar all the laws and regulations that the FDA has created with reference to gluten and allergens will be available.

I'm going to try and make it as simple as possible. Following is a list of things that could be on the label or ingredients list that definitely contain gluten and some items that might have gluten in them. Also remember that wheat free does not mean gluten free. There is also a list of gluten free foods.

List Of Foods To Avoid

Barley (flakes, flour, pearl)

Brewers yeast

Bulgur (Parboiled wheat groats, most often Durum wheat)

Couscous (steamed tiny balls of crushed durum wheat semolina)

Durum wheat

Einkor

Emmer

Farina (milled wheat served as a cereal)

Farro

Gliadin

Graham flour (coarsely ground, unsifted flour including the germ and bran)

Kamut

Malt (cereal grains which are germinated, then the germination process is halted by drying)

Malt Extract

Malt Syrup (unrefined sweetener made from malt)

Malt Vinegar

Malted Milk (powdered gruel made from mixture of malted   barley, wheat flour and evaporated whole milk)

Matzo (unleavened bread made from grain)

Rye

Seitan (wheat gluten)

Semolina (coarse, purified wheat middlings of durum wheat mainly used in making pasta and couscous)

Spelt

Triticale (hybrid of wheat and rye)

Wheat Bran

Wheat Flour

Wheat Germ

Wheat Starch

Things That May Contain Gluten, Ensure To Read The Label

Artificial Colours or Flavouring

Baking Powder

Beer and some Alcohols (safe ones listed later)

Candy (may be dusted with wheat flour)

Canned Soups and Boxed Soups (not all)

Caramel Colours or Flavouring

Cheese Spreads and some processed cheese (not all)

Chocolate (may contain malt flavouring)

Dextrin (may be derived from wheat)

Dip Mixes

Dry sauce mixes and gravies

Extenders and Binders

French fries

Ice Cream and Frozen Yoghurt (some flavours contain gluten so ensure you read the label)

Mayonnaise

Mustard (some are gluten free, listed later)

Nuts, dusted or roasted

Processed meats, Cold cuts, Sausages, Hot Dogs

Salad Dressing

Sour Cream

Vinegar, malt or non-distilled

Other Items That Are Not Food

Cosmetics
Hairspray
Lipstick
Medications

Mouthwash

Play dough

Shampoos

 Vitamins

Remember that some of these items may be gluten free if listed as such, but please read the labels on everything, **DONT ASSUME** anything. We can all be contaminated at some time or another. Even as I sit here writing this book, I have been sick for a couple of weeks with all the old symptoms that I used to get. I was having the hardest time trying to figure out what was causing my belly to look like a balloon and feel this pain and all this turmoil again. I finally found the item that was causing me the problem - it was one of my vitamins (*wow*). My husband usually gets all the vitamins for us and we always get the same kind but this time he forgot to look on the back and he ASSUMED they were still the same and so did I. Lesson learned for both of us and now I must wait for the turmoil in my body to calm, which could take some time. This is an example of how easy it is to be caught. We can all make a mistake, especially in the beginning, so don't be hard on yourself. Make sure you listen to the messages your body is always sending you. You have to listen to what your body is saying to acquire optimal health.

List Of Foods That Are Gluten Free

Fruit

Acai

Apples

Apricot

Bananas

Blackberries

Blueberries

Cantaloupe

Cherries

Coconut

Cranberries

Currants

Dates

Figs

Grapefruit

Grapes

Guava

Honeydew Melons

Huckleberries

Kiwi

Kumquat

Lemons

Limes

Mandarins

Mangoes

Mulberries

Nectarines

Oranges

Papaya

Passion Fruit

Peaches

Pears

Persimmons

Pineapples

Plantain

Plums

Quince

Raspberries

Strawberries

Tangerines

Watermelons

Vegetables, Legumes And Beans

Acorn

Agar

Alfalfa

Algae

Amaranth

Arrowroot

Artichoke

Arugula

Asparagus

Avocado

Bamboo Shoots

Beans

Beans, Green and Yellow

Bell Peppers

Bok Choi

Broccoli

Brussel Sprouts

Cabbage

Carob

Carrots

Cauliflower

Celery

Chard

Chives

Collard Greens

Corn

Cucumber

Eggplant

Endive

Fennel

Fiddleheads

Garlic

Kale

Kohlrabi

Leeks

Lentils

Lettuce

Mushrooms

Okra

Onions

Parsley

Parsnips

Peas, All

Peppers

Potato, All

Pumpkin

Radish

Rutabaga

Seaweed

Spinach

Squash, All

Tomato

Turnips

Watercress

Zucchini

Flours And Grains

Almond Flour

Amaranth Flour

Amaranth, grain or leaf

Arrowroot

Bean flour

Besan also known as Gram or Chick Pea Flour

Brown Rice

Brown Rice Flour

Buckwheat

Buckwheat Flour

Cassava (Tapioca)

Coconut Flour

Corn Meal

Corn Starch

Cotton Seed

Flax Seed (Ground)

Millet

Oat Flour (that is gluten-free)

Oats (that are gluten-free)

Pea Flour

Potato Flour

Potato Starch

Quinoa

Quinoa Flour

Rice, All

Sago Starch

Sorghum

Sorghum Flour

Soy Flour

Tapioca Flour (Tapioca Starch)

Teff

Teff Flour

Yeast

Yucca Flour

Egg And Dairy Products

Butter

Casein

Cheese, All

Cream

Eggs

Sour Cream

Whey

Yoghurt

Meat

All Wild Game

Alligator

Beef

Buffalo

Chicken

Duck

Goat

Quail

Rabbit

Snake

Turkey

Veal

Venison

Herbs and Spices

Anise

Basil

Caraway

Chamomile

Cilantro

Coriander

Dill

Fennel

Lavender

Lemon Grass

Marjoram

Oregano

Parsley

Rosemary

Sage

Thyme

Other Items

Alcohol that has been distilled (such as vodka, tequila gin) and most wine is safe

Baking Soda

Honey

Jams

Juice

Mustard is considered safe (Annie's Naturals – all types, French's, Heinz, Koop's, Organicville, Gulden's)

Nuts (not dusted or roasted)

Oils

Seeds

Syrup

Vanilla Extract, Real or Artificial (If concerned that it might not be safe you can use McCormick's, Club House, Kirkland, but because vanilla extracts, both natural and artificial, contain pure distilled alcohol they should all be gluten-free)

Vinegars are considered safe (Apple cider, Wine vinegar, Cane vinegar)

Vitamins, most (Read the label, some use flour for humidity control and as a filler)

Xanthan gum

Chapter 7

Celiac Disease Symptoms

In this chapter I am going to list the most common symptoms that children and adults with celiac disease experience as well as some of my own experiences. As this chapter is read remember that just because you have or don't have some of these symptoms it does not mean that you have celiac disease. The only way to know for certain is to be tested as discussed in chapter 4. Also remember that many of these symptoms will also appear if you have gluten intolerance or a Wheat Allergy.

After reading this chapter you may feel that you have some answers to some of the problems you may be experiencing. But remember it requires a doctor to make a diagnosis. Just keep in mind that the content in this chapter and in Chapter #8 may feel unexciting but may shed light on something pertaining to your life. Feel free to just skim through but don't let this stop you from making sure you reap the benefits of Chapter #9, Your Future Looks Brighter.

Symptoms of Celiac Disease

Abdominal cramps

Abdominal pain

Anemia

Bloating or Swollen Belly

Bone or Joint Pain

Canker Sores

Constipation

Depression or Anxiety

Dermatitis Herpetiformis

Diarrhea

Fatty Stool or Foul-Smelling Flatulence or Gas

Headaches

Infertility

Miscarriages

Missed Menstrual Periods

Early Menopause

Nausea

Numbness and Tingling in hands or feet
(Raynaud Phenomenon)

Seizures

Ulcers or Sores on stomach or lining of intestines

Symptoms That Usually Only Occur In Children

Delay in Puberty

Failure to Thrive

Slowed Growth

Weight Loss

Symptoms Of A Wheat Allergy

Anaphylaxis

Cramps

Diarrhea

Difficulty Breathing

Headaches

Hives, Itchy Rash or Swelling of the Skin

Itchy, Watery Eyes

Nasal Congestion

Swelling, Itching or Irritation of Mouth and Throat

Vomiting or Nausea

As can be seen some of these symptoms can be the same or similar to the symptoms of celiac disease. There are some big differences such as a wheat allergy causing a life-threatening reaction called anaphylaxis, which means you have to carry an Epi pen (Epinephrine auto injector) with you at all times. Also, if you have a wheat allergy you may still be able to eat things like barley or rye.

Symptoms of Gluten Intolerance

Abdominal Cramps

Abdominal Pain

Anemia

Bloating

Bone or Joint Pain

Canker Sores

Constipation

Depression or Anxiety

Dermatitis (Herpetiformis)

Diarrhea

Fatty Stool or Foul-Smelling Stool

Gas (Flatulence)

Headaches

Infertility, Miscarriages

Missed Periods, Menopause

Nausea

Numbness or Tingling in hands and feet
(Raynaud's Phenomenon)

Seizures

Tiredness

Ulcers or sores on Stomach or Lining of Intestines

Once again, some of these symptoms are similar to those experienced by people with celiac disease or a wheat allergy. Therefore, it is hard to know exactly which one you may be experiencing without being tested. This is why it's important to get tested so that you don't keep damaging your intestines or putting yourself in life threatening situations. In the next part of this chapter I will explain the symptoms of celiac disease and hope that you will better understand what they are.

Abdominal Cramps

This is when sharp pains are felt in the abdominal area - which is located between the chest and groin. This is caused by contractions of the muscles. The pain could last minutes or just a few seconds. *I often experienced sharp pains, feeling like knives trying to come out of my abdominal area and it would move around like it was gas pains. I always felt that if I could just pass some gas, I would get some relief, but passing gas was always very rare.*

Abdominal pain

This is when there are painful sensations in the abdominal area, again it is located between the chest and the groin. You may hear this referred to as a tummy ache, belly ache or stomach ache.

Anemia

This is a condition in which the red blood cell count is lower than it should be. Red blood cells carry oxygen from the lungs to the cells that make up the body. Anemia is normally caused by a lack of iron (which captures and carries the oxygen in the red blood cells) and B12 (folic acid) usually causing weakness, tiredness, and faintness - also you will look pale due to the lack of red blood cells. This can be the result of the body not absorbing nutrients because the small intestine villi have been damaged by celiac disease.

Over time the red blood cells will go back to normal provided you take positive steps to live a gluten free life style. Of course, there may be other reasons for the Anemia so ensure other   possibilities are ruled out. Doctors will order a hemoglobin test (Hemoglobin is the iron-containing oxygen-transport metalloprotein in the red blood cells of all vertebrates) because they are measuring the ability of blood to transport oxygen, which relates back to the number of red blood cells. *Anemia is something I suffered from for many of years. It was only resolved after I went on a gluten free diet.*

Bloating

In this condition gas, irregular swelling and increased size of the abdominal area (between the groin and the chest) is experienced. This can sometimes be painful and cause a feeling of being full. It is also known as Intestinal Inflammation and is triggered by something you have eaten. Bloating could also be a sign of constipation or a partial or completely impacted intestine. *This is something I have suffered with for my whole life. It was the main reason I always saw myself as being overweight. Even when gluten was eliminated from my diet, I was still experiencing bloating and inflammation. It wasn't until I eliminated dairy, corn, sugar and a few other foods that I started knowing what normal felt like. I still have to make sure I keep listening to my body because it is always sending me messages.*

Bone and Joint Pain

Bone and joint pain are sometimes caused by the body experiencing inflammation, which could be a reaction to gluten. It could also be caused by other foods, osteoporosis or arthritis which will be explained in the next chapter.

Canker Sores

These are small ulcers on the inside of the mouth, tongue, lips or throat and they can be very painful. Canker sores can also be caused by vitamin deficiencies, autoimmune disorders, spicy or acidic foods, hormones and stress.

Constipation

This is when a person passes fewer than 3 stools a week. It is also when the stool is hard or lumpy and the person is having a difficult time passing it. It can also be very painful and there is usually bloating in the abdomen due to the buildup of waste.

I would like to share a story that was an awkward situation. The doctor had put me on some antibiotics to clear up an infection I had been struggling with. I started experiencing a lot of different side effects to the drug prescribed. I was experiencing extreme bloating that made me feel and look like I was 9 months pregnant, diarrhea, nausea and a severe headache. This went on for about a week before I went to see the doctor.

The doctor was concerned that the bloating was extreme and sent me right to the hospital to have an x-ray done. The results from the x-ray showed that I was full of stool. I was shocked. How could this be true considering all the watery stool I was experiencing (diarrhea) several times a day. I also felt confused because my diet consisted of all fruits, vegetables, gluten free foods and no meat, dairy or eggs. I was living a healthy whole food plant-based lifestyle. I soon learned that you could still have a partially impacted bowel. This is when there is still some stool passing by the partial obstruction.

Bowel obstructions occur when a mass of hard dry stool is unable to pass through the colon or rectum. This is a serious issue if not treated and could be life threatening.

My almost completely impacted stool was in the upper intestines. I spent the next couple weeks following the doctor's strict instructions, which was supposed to help break it up. This wasn't working so there were more trips to the doctor and hospital for a variety of different tests. This was to make sure that it wasn't anything really serious. After a couple of months of still having some problems I went for a colonoscopy. And I was privileged to spend the 2 days before with no food and an intense bowel cleanse. After the procedure the doctor put me on a 3-month diet of high fibre and evening laxatives. Because of the problem I have with gluten it was more challenging to find things that were gluten free and more natural. If you are interested in some of the steps and foods, I used to help improve my health refer to chapter #9 Your Future Looks Brighter.

So, the point I am trying to make by sharing this learning adventure I was put though is to show that you could be constipated and still be passing a very watery stool. Extreme bloating would be a good sign that this might be happening. I think this has possibly been a contributor to some of my intense bloating experiences (How crazy is that).

Depression and Anxiety

Depression

Depression is something many people go though and can sometimes become a serious mood disorder. It affects how people feel, think and handle daily activities. There could be a number of reasons why depression is being experienced. It could just be going though the tough time trying to find out what is wrong. Depression could happen after finding out that you have celiac disease, wheat intolerance or allergies, and now realizing the challenging, lifelong journey ahead. Depression could also be caused by malabsorption of the nutrients the brain needs to function properly. Depression can also be caused by an inflammation response to the gluten that might be affecting the body. But it won't last forever because once you find out and start making the necessary changes you will feel an amazing transformation, just be patient.

I know how hard depression can be, I suffered from it for too many years. I remember that the more times I was told by doctors that there was nothing wrong and that it was all psychological the more depressed I would get. It affected everything I did and all my relationships. It also kept me from living a life of happiness, love and peace. And my dreams were not being fulfilled. Another thing to keep in mind is that there are many other things in our lives that can cause depression and we don't have to go though it alone. You should seek support or medical attention especially if you have thoughts of suicide or death. No one should ever have to feel this way.

Signs and Symptoms of Depression

Aches and pain

Decreased energy or Fatigue

Difficulty concentrating, Remembering and Making decisions

Difficulty sleeping or Oversleeping

Digestive problems

Headaches

Helplessness

Hopelessness

Irritability

Sadness

Thoughts of suicide or Death

Weight changes and/or Appetite changes

Anxiety

Anxiety, is a condition that may affect many people at sometime or another in their lives and can be caused by many things other then celiac disease.

Symptoms of Anxiety

Excessive worry

Fear of an outcome

Inner turmoil

Nervousness

Overwhelming emotions

Racing heartbeat

Dermatitis Herpetiformis

Dermatitis Herpetiformis is usually caused by an intolerance or allergy to gluten. It's also sometimes called celiac disease of the skin. They both have the IgA antibody present and that is caused by stimulation of the immune system by gluten. This causes serious inflammation of the skin, which will appear red and swollen. There will also be small blisters that are painful. The blisters will usually appear on the knees, elbows and buttocks, but may also appear on the back, shoulders, scalp and face. It may take a couple of years to see a complete change because even a trace could cause it to flare up again. It is said that about 20% of people with Dermatitis Herpetiformis have normal small intestine biopsies - this is because Gluten doesn't affect everyone's body in the same way, only the inflammation part is the same.

Diarrhea

Diarrhea is when bowel movements (feces) are loose and watery and occur three or more times a day. Diarrhea is a common symptom of celiac disease although it may only occur occasionally. There are many other things that can cause diarrhea such as digestive disorders, lactose intolerance, bacterial infections and parasites, food poisoning, viruses, flu, medications, antibiotics and many others. If diarrhea persists for more then 3 days in adults or 24 hours in children and includes some of the side effects listed below seek medical attention. Of course, there are many side effects that come from having diarrhea which include.

Symptoms of Diarrhea

Abdominal pain

Bloody stool

Chills & fever

Cramping

Nausea

Urgent use of the bathroom

Fatty stool (Steatorrhea)

Fatty stool is a term used to describe bowel movements that contain gobs of fat and are loose and floating. The bowel movement will look slimy or oily. It will possibly be grey to pale yellow in colour and will most likely be floating. It will also probably be very foul smelling. Fatty stools usually occur because of a problem absorbing fats and nutrients through the intestinal lining. Fatty stool can be caused by many digestive absorption problems like Crohn's disease, leaky gut, Whipple disease, lactose intolerance, fatty foods and celiac disease, as well as pancreatic, liver and gallbladder problems.

[56]

This was something in my life that I thought was quite normal - floating stools that were foul smelling and oily looking. But it is not normal. If you have it consult with a doctor so you can find cause.

Flatulence

Flatulence is more commonly called a fart. Flatulence is a build up of gas in the stomach, bowels or intestines. When the body is working properly gas is passed though the intestines and colon through contractions of the muscles. There are many things that cause gas besides celiac disease. Different foods being the most common. Here are just a few examples: beans, lentils, broccoli, cauliflower, cabbage, onion and many more. And they don't all have the same affect on everyone. As well digestive problems in general can cause gas. *This was a very painful thing for me, I think mostly because I couldn't pass it. I would feel like there was something alive inside me that couldn't find its way out. It was experienced as a very sharp pain or just unbearable pressure.*

Headache

While most of us have experienced a headache at some time or another, someone with celiac disease may be more prone to having headaches. A headache could be a sharp pain, a throbbing or a dull pain and could be anywhere in the head or upper neck. There are many things that could cause a headache like allergies, environmental issues, food, illnesses, stress, tension and many more.

Infertility and Pregnancy

Infertility (inability to conceive children) and problems with pregnancy have been suggested as a possible link to celiac disease. When someone who has celiac disease is not strictly following a gluten free diet they will be suffering from malabsorption of folic acid and other nutrients. This could be part of the cause of the inability to conceive, as well as the reasons for miscarriage, a stillborn or premature baby or a baby with low birth weight. There could be other reasons such as a disruption of a normal immune system. This is something I know first hand but only discovered long after the birth of my little miracle. I have shared my story in chapter #10.

Menstrual Periods and Menopause

It is thought that in some women there could be a link between menstrual disorders and early onset menopause. Normal menstrual periods are approximately 28 days. It is the body's way of going though a series of changes to prepare the uterus for pregnancy. When menstrual periods are not normal it is very frustrating. Periods may be late, or early, or just not consistent as to when it is coming. It can be related to painful periods or Endometriosis which I will share with you in the next chapter. It can also be the reason for lateness of the first period. Menopause should naturally occur around age 50 but early or premature menopause is referred to as happening before age 40. Premature menopause can be caused by an autoimmune disease.

I certainly had my experiences with abnormal periods, and many trips to the doctors, only to be told that there was nothing wrong. In my mid 30s, I had one doctor suggest that maybe I had endometriosis and wanted to put me though some tests (I felt they were more experiments than tests because he didn't explain the purpose properly). He wanted to give me a needle (Lupron) that would put me into a simulated early menopause. If the drug did what the doctor suspected it would, then he would proceed with testing for endometriosis.

After my husband and I read all the side effects of this drug, as well as reading up on what other doctors were saying about how dangerous this drug was, I decided not to use it. That was enough information for me to make my final decision. Not long after that I started premenopausal symptoms, which happened in my late 30s (which I felt was way too young), but I was grateful that I finally had no more periods.

I also was experiencing some problems with bladder control while I was premenopausal and I would like to share my story. I hope for your sake you don't relate but if you do, you're not alone. I had just finished shopping and was loading my car with the groceries when I had to go pee. I tried to hold it in but it just let go right there in the parking lot. I broke down and started to cry. I laid some plastic bags on the seats and drove home. I was feeling embarrassed and sorry for myself. But this was what I needed to push me to make an appointment to go see the doctor. The doctor ended up putting me on menopausal hormone replacement therapy after I shared everything that was going on and controlling my life in every aspect. Wow, did this ever help with some of my many problems.

Symptoms of Perimenopause

No periods for 1yr

Bladder control problems

Changes in sexual desire

Changes in emotions (mood swings)

Changes in menstrual periods

Hot flashes

Longer and longer intervals between menstrual periods

Night sweats

Painful intercourse

Spotting or heavy bleeding when you do have a period

Vaginal dryness

You may only have a few symptoms, but one thing is for sure, you will not have a period when you are in full menopause.

Nausea

Nausea is a very uncomfortable feeling in the stomach that feels like you are going to vomit, but most times you don't. That uncomfortable feeling just continues in the stomach. Nausea can be caused by many things like stomach flu, medication, motion sickness, some diseases and of course, food. This is the body's way of saying "I don't think we should be eating this." But most of us haven't learned to listen to our body and even when we are listening, we ignore it because we think it's too hard to change or we just don't want to give up what it is causing the nausea. This is because instant gratification can outweigh what might happen later and our brains only like to think about what brings us immediate pleasure. This is a hard thing for the brain to overcome. But I know you can do it - because I did.

Numbness and Tingling In The Hands and Feet

Numbness and tingling in the hands and feet can be caused by nerve damage - a condition called Peripheral Neuropathy. Peripheral Neuropathy can be the result of vitamin deficiency and inflammation that can occur in someone with untreated celiac disease. There are also other things that could be the reason for this condition, such as diabetes, autoimmune diseases, kidney failure, alcoholism, herniated discs, and medications. Numbness and tingling in the toes and fingers are also a symptom of Raynaud's phenomenon which I will discuss in the next chapter.

Seizures

Seizures, are uncontrolled or sudden involuntary movements of the body due to abnormal electrical activity in the brain. Having untreated celiac disease, which causes malnourishment and inflammation, can affect the brain (leaky brain). There is also a link between gut flora (bacteria) and the brain. Seizures can also be caused by many other things such as epilepsy, abnormal levels of sodium, magnesium, calcium, or glucose (diabetes) and most autoimmune diseases about which I will give more information in my next chapter.

Ulcers or Sores

Ulcers are sores that normally occur on the stomach lining or the lining of the intestines and are also referred to as canker sores when they occur in the mouth. Canker sores occur mainly on the inside of your cheeks and lips. They are red with a white or yellow center and are painful. It is said that most ulcers in the stomach are caused by taking aspirin and ibuprofen for a long period of time. Also, consuming alcohol and smoking makes it worse. A gluten free diet may help prevent ulcers in the digestive system. Elimination of gluten could be one of the things that alleviate an ulcer.

Symptoms of Ulcers

Dull pain or Soreness

Burning in the stomach

These Are Complications That Usually Occur In Children

Delay in puberty

Delay in puberty is when there is a delay in the physical development to adulthood. This is when there haven't been any changes in a girl's body such as breast development, pubic hair growth and starting menstrual periods until later then 13 years of age. In boys it is when the enlargement of testicles and the penis, growth of pubic hair and voice change occurs later then 14 years of age.

Slowed Growth, Failure To Thrive

Failure to thrive in children is when the child is not reaching the height and weight on the standard growth charts for their age. It is usually a sign that the child is suffering from one of or some of the following - undernourished, has an illness, an eating disorder, Gastroesophageal Reflex Disease (GERD), chronic diarrhea, cystic fibrosis and/or of course celiac disease.

Weight Loss

Weight loss could be a sign that your child is not getting the nutrition they need. This could be the reason why they have lost weight, but remember there are a lot of other things that cause weight loss besides not getting the correct nutrition.

CHAPTER 8

CONDITIONS RELATED TO CELIAC DISEASE

This chapter lists some of the many conditions that are possibly related to celiac disease. This means that if you have one of these conditions you may be at higher risk of having or developing celiac disease, or if you have celiac disease you may be at higher risk of developing one of these related conditions. There may also be no risk at all, especially if you are eating a gluten free diet.

Once one autoimmune disease has been diagnosed there is a higher risk of getting another autoimmune disease. The immune system is supposed to protect the body from disease and harm, but if you have an autoimmune disease the body's immune system mistakes healthy cells for intruders and will attack its own body cells. Once the immune system is attacking one area of the body it is possible it will make this mistake again and attack a different area of the body.

There are more and more studies linking inflammation and autoimmune diseases. Inflammation in the body is most often caused by something that is being eaten. Examples are: gluten, corn sugar, dairy, fats (oils) and even meats. The body may be sensitive or allergic to one or more of these foods.

There are some great books available that I recommend reading to better understand some different doctors' thoughts on the studies relating to the connections between autoimmune diseases and food, and some of the data from the studies that they used. Some of them are: *The Autoimmune Fix by Tom O'Brian, The China Study by T. Colin Campbell and his son Dr. Thomas Campbell, The Longevity Plan by Dr. John Day and Jane Ann Day, and Cure Your Child with Food by Kelly Dorfman, MS, LND.* I will list more at the back of the book. Please note that some of these are controversial because of methodology and/or lack of supporting studies.

List of Conditions Related To Celiac Disease

Addison's Disease & Adrenal Insufficiency

Arthritis

Asthma

Attention Deficit Hyperactive Disorder (ADHD)

Autism

Cancers

Candida

Casein Allergy

Cognitive Impairment

Crohn's Disease

Diabetes

Down Syndrome

Dyspepsia and Acid Reflux

Eczema

Epilepsy

Fibromyalgia

Heart Burn

Irritable Bowel Syndrome (IBS)

Kidney Disease

Lactose Intolerance

Liver Disease

Lupus

Migraines

Multiple Sclerosis

Myasthenia

Osteoporosis

Psoriasis

Raynaud's Phenomena

Sarcoidosis

Schizophrenia

Scleroderma

Sepsis

Sjogren's Syndrome

Thrombocytopenic (Low Platelets)

Thyroid Pancreatic and Hashimoto Disease

Tuberculosis

Turner Syndrome

Ulcerative Colitis

Vitiligo

Williams Syndrome

Brief Description of Conditions Related to Celiac Disease

Addison's Disease

Addison's Disease, also called Adrenal Insufficiency, occurs when there is low hormone production by the adrenal glands. Addison's usually occurs when there has been some damage to the adrenal gland. The adrenal gland produces steroid hormones called cortisol, aldosterone and the hormone adrenaline. These hormones help regulate blood pressure and help with the way digested food is metabolized for energy. As well it helps with the way stress is handled. Our bodies also use the adrenal hormones (DHEA) to make the male sex hormone androgen and the female sex hormone estrogen. Cortisol has other important jobs as well. It slows the inflammatory response of the immune system which is the way the body defends itself from harmful substances, viruses and bacteria. It also aids in heart and blood vessel maintenance. Addison's Disease is considered to be an autoimmune disease.

Common Symptoms of Addison's Disease

Abdominal pain

Long lasting fatigue

Loss of appetite

Weight loss

Other Symptoms

Craving for salty foods

Diarrhea

Headache

Irregular or absent menstrual periods

Irritability and depression

Low interest in sex in women

Low blood sugar

Low blood pressure

Nausea

Sweating

Vomiting

Arthritis

Arthritis is a term often used to mean any disorder of the joints. There are over 100 types of arthritis but the two main types are osteoarthritis, which is degenerative, and rheumatoid arthritis which is an autoimmune disease in which the immune system attacks the cartilage and lining of the joints. It may attack only one or multiple joints. Eating foods that cause inflammation only adds to the pain of this condition.

Symptoms of Arthritis

Joint pain

Stiffness

Inflammation of joints

Asthma

Asthma is a lung Disease in which the airways narrow and swell and produce extra mucus making it difficult to breathe. This can trigger coughing, wheezing and shortness of breath. Asthma cannot be cured but it can be controlled.

Symptoms of Asthma

Chest tightness

Coughing

Shortness of breath

Wheezing

Attention Deficit Hyperactivity Disorder (ADHD)

Attention Deficit Hyperactivity Disorder (ADHD) is a brain disorder found mainly in children, although it may also be found in adults. In this condition difficulty keeping focus, disorganized thoughts, excessive fidgeting, tapping or talking, as well as being very impulsive are some of the main symptoms. These symptoms may be present in all of us, but if they are caused by ADHD these symptoms will be more severe and more frequent.

A possible association between celiac disease and ADHD has been reported, with significant improvement in behaviour when on a gluten free diet in some cases. The link between gluten and behavioural problems in children with celiac disease is well documented. Some studies are also finding

[67]

that any foods that may be causing inflammation can contribute to this condition. It might be worth a try to eliminate gluten if you suspect it is causing inflammation. What do you have to lose? Nothing but wheat.

Symptoms of Attention Deficit Hyperactivity Disorder

Inattention (paying attention)

Hyperactivity (trouble sitting)

Impulsivity (acting before thinking)

Autism

Autism Spectrum Disorder is a brain disorder that affects social interaction and communication with others. One of its primary symptoms is repetitive behaviour. It is usually detected in young children. Some people with autism experience gastrointestinal disturbances. I know a couple of friends that put their children on a completely gluten free, sugar free and casein free diet and their autistic child showed many improvements, not just with their gastrointestinal disturbances, but also with improved behaviour and the communication symptoms of autism. This may be worth a try - especially if the child is still young - because the older they get the harder it is to get them to change their routine. It can still be done when they are older, it is just more difficult.

Symptoms of Autism

Don't like change

Like following a set routine

Have trouble listening or looking at others

Having unusual behaviours that they repeat

Interests that they overly focus on

These are just a few of the most common symptoms - there are many more

Cancer

Cancer is a disease that can affect any part of the body. The body is made up of trillions of cells and cancer starts at the cellular level. Normal cells have specific functions in the body and cancer hijacks these cells, making them reproduce uncontrollably, do things that they are not supposed to, or move to locations where they are not supposed to be. Because they continue to divide without knowing when to stop, they can form growths called tumours. There are a couple of cancers that someone with untreated celiac disease may be at a slightly higher risk of developing than someone in good health. These cancers are Hodgkin's lymphoma and non-Hodgkin's lymphoma. These are blood cancers affecting the immune system. There are a few reasons why someone with untreated celiac disease has an increased risk of developing cancer. One is the continuous inflammation the body is experiencing; another is because the body is trying to focus on fighting so it can destroy the intruder - gluten. It could also be a damaged, leaky gut that is allowing the toxins and carcinogens to be absorbed into the body. It could also be caused by malnutrition due to having celiac disease

General Symptoms of Cancer

Enlarged lymph nodes

Swollen abdominal area or pain

Weight loss

Fever

Chest pain

Breathing problems

Coughing

Candida Albicans

Candida is a yeast or fungus. When this yeast or fungus grows out of control it can cause an infection in the intestinal tract, vagina or mouth. If your body's immune system is not working right it will be hard to control the growth of these yeasts and once there is an overgrowth happening it can cause the onset of many problems.

Until I eliminated Gluten, I had a continuous yeast infection. I just could not get it under control, no matter what I did. I was using prescription and non-prescription drugs, as well as herbal remedies and nothing seemed to work. After my 40th birthday I finally started to understand why I could not get it under control because I had educated myself and taken control of my life once and for all. When I eliminated gluten, things did get much better, but still not perfect. I still would have the occasional infection. But then I removed almost all sugar as well as most processed foods. The yeast infections went away for good once I had removed the foods responsible and this is when I started to feel amazing.

There are a lot of other things that can cause yeast infections. You are welcome to try what I did - it might work for you as well. Most people don't want to change their diet, but I had no choice. If you haven't found something that works for you consider the possibility that it may be the food you are eating. There are many symptoms and they will vary depending on whether it is in the throat, vagina or intestinal tract.

Symptoms of Candida (Yeast Infection)

Vaginal Yeast Infection

Burning pain during Intercourse

Itching, pain and Irritation in and around the vagina

Vaginal discharge

Vaginal rash

Intestinal Yeast Overgrowth

Bloating, cramping, gas

Diarrhea, constipation

Food allergies

Headaches

Irritability

Digestive problems

Weak immune system

Oral Thrush

White patches or dots on the inside of the mouth, tongue and roof

or side of the mouth

Redness in the throat and mouth

Loss of taste

Burning or slight pain in the mouth

Casein Allergy

Casein is a protein found in dairy products and lactose is the sugar found in dairy. Although both of them can cause difficulty with digestion a casein allergy is life threatening because the body produces histamines that will cause breathing passages to swell and close. Lactose intolerance will be covered separately because although it can be debilitating, it is not as immediately life threatening as an allergy. If you have celiac disease you may not be able to consume dairy products because of the inability to digest food properly. It is quite possible that after going gluten free and giving the body some time to heal, you may be able to consume dairy once again.

I have never been able to enjoy dairy again so I have had to keep it out of my diet. There are some awesome alternatives and I feel that they are healthier choices. Some examples are: rice, almonds, coconuts, cashew and soy milks and cheeses.

Symptoms of Casein Allergy

Swelling of lips, mouth, and tongue

Nasal congestion

Runny nose

Itchy eyes

Wheezing, coughing

Itchy skin

Rash or hives

Mild Cognitive Impairment

Mild cognitive impairment is a condition in which the brain has trouble with memory or problem solving (thinking skills) functions relative to the age of the individual. This also will increase the risk of Alzheimer's and dementia in the future. All these brain conditions have some links to inflammation in the brain and, as explained earlier, celiac disease can cause inflammation anywhere in the body. This is one reason to control inflammation - so there will be no suffering from any problems relating to the brain.

Symptoms of Mild Cognitive Impairment

Forgetting things, a lot more, such as appointments

Having difficulty finding your way around familiar places

Having trouble making decisions

Having trouble understanding simple instructions

Family and friends are starting to notice that you are having trouble   with the above list

Crohn's Disease

Crohn's Disease is a bowel disease that causes the digestive tract to be irritated and inflamed. Any part of the digestive system can be affected by Crohn's Disease.

Crohn's disease is not well understood and there are environmental, immune and bacterial factors in genetically susceptible individuals.

Symptoms of Crohn's Disease

Diarrhea

Abdominal pain and cramping

Weight loss

Nausea

Anemia

Fever

Stress has been known to make the symptoms much worse

Diabetes

Diabetes is when the blood glucose (blood sugar) level is too high. The body produces insulin which helps the sugar in food to be delivered to the cells and used for energy. There are three types of diabetes - Type 1, Type 2, and Gestational diabetes.

Type 1 is an autoimmune disease in which the body has destroyed the insulin producing cells in the pancreas, which results in no insulin production at all. Remember, having one autoimmune disease increases the risk of getting or having another. Needles will have to be taken every day to provide the required insulin.

Type 2 is when the body is not making enough insulin or not using it well, and help is required to provide the body with the extra it needs or help to use what is there correctly.

Gestational Diabetes occurs during pregnancy and is similar to type 2 diabetes. It is caused by hormonal changes or life style.

It is estimated (at the time I am writing this book) that over 400 million people are living with diabetes, and almost half of them are undiagnosed. And approximately 8 to 10% of the

400 million will develop celiac disease.

Symptoms of Type 1 diabetes appear quickly while the symptoms of Type 2 take longer to develop.

Symptoms of Diabetes

Frequent urination

Increased thirst

Increased hunger

Blurred vision

Fatigue

Numbness in feet or hands

Unexplained weight loss

Sores that don't heal

Down Syndrome

Down Syndrome is a genetic disorder that occurs when a child is born with an extra copy (full or partial) of chromosome 21. This will cause mild to moderate intellectual disability and delay in physical development, as well as the display of characteristic facial features. There is a chance that if you have Down Syndrome you may have digestion problems or celiac disease. Someone with Down Syndrome will also have a harder time expressing problems with digestion so they should be screened for celiac disease.

Symptoms of Down Syndrome

Poor immune function

Physical and intellectual disabilities

Increased number of other health problems

Hearing and vision disorders

Slower growth

Many more symptoms such as susceptibilities to some cancers and congenital heart disease

Dyspepsia (Indigestion)

Indigestion is a condition in which digestion of food causes pain, bloating, excessive gas and numerous other symptoms, usually because of something eaten or eating too quickly. Indigestion is a problem most people will experience at one time or another and most people who have celiac disease can improve their chances of not having Indigestion by eating a gluten free diet.

Symptoms of Indigestion

Feeling full

Upper abdominal pain

Bloating

Belching

Nausea

Eczema

Eczema is a group of diseases that cause inflammation of the skin. It is also called dermatitis which I discuss in chapter 7. It appears approximately 3 times more often in individuals with celiac disease and twice as often in relatives of those with celiac disease.

I remember as a child always struggling with eczema. It was mainly on my face and arms so as a child I was always trying to hide it. The doctor would give my Mom suggestions about what they thought could be causing it but no one ever considered the possibility of gluten, even though I had so many other things that could have been related to celiac disease. That's why I'm so grateful that doctors are much more aware of it now. Because of this many children and adults will not have to suffer from skin problems - if it can be fixed with something as simple as diet.

Symptoms of Eczema

Rough red bumpy skin

Dry and itchy skin

Inflamed blisters that can become crusty, thick and scaly

Epilepsy

Epilepsy is when normal neuronal functions in the brain are disrupted. When this happens, it can cause a seizure. The common causes of epilepsy are trauma to the brain, stroke and brain tumours. Epilepsy can sometimes be controlled with medicines, surgery and through diet. This is where the connection to celiac disease comes in. Some people can control it when they eliminate gluten.

When I was in my late teens and 20's I had many seizures. It wasn't until I was in my 40's that I found that there was a possible link between celiac disease and epilepsy. It worked for me – no gluten, no more seizures.

Symptom of Epilepsy

Unusual sensations

Unusual emotions

Body movements such as muscle spasms and convulsions

Loss of consciousness

Fibromyalgia Syndrome

Fibromyalgia Syndrome is a chronic condition with widespread pain affecting the muscles and soft tissues. The chronic pain of this condition affects day to day activities. There is no real link between celiac disease and fibromyalgia but diet has helped many of people suffering with this. Non-celiac gluten sensitivity (NCGS) may be an underlying cause of fibromyalgia symptoms (further research is needed) - thus the elimination of gluten has worked for some, even though they do not have celiac disease. If it could stop the chronic pain it would certainly be worth trying because I know you would like to be able to take control of your life again. It is estimated that around 9% of people with celiac disease were originally diagnosed with fibromyalgia.

Symptoms of Fibromyalgia

Muscle pain

Sleep problems

Fatigue

Memory and mood problems

Chronic pain

GI Symptoms such as acid reflux

Non-Ulcer Dyspepsia

Heart Burn

Heart Burn is a form of indigestion in which gastric acid is regurgitated back up into the esophagus. I would like to share an interesting story with you.

I was having a lot of problem with chest pains, and sometimes they were very severe. I remember my husband and I were on one of our yearly snowmobile trips and we had just finished lunch. We started back out on the trail, which of course is in the middle of nowhere, and I had to stop because I thought I was having a heart attack. I took some aspirin, laid on the back of my seat and waited in pain until I felt like I couldn't even move from the position I was in. Of course, back then I didn't like going to the doctor because I felt they never found anything and would always tell me it was all in my head.

Years later my father died of a massive heart attack just after I had started my journey to find out what was really causing my digestive problems. Because I had no other symptoms related to heart burn, I thought I should get these chest pains looked at, considering my family history. To make a long story short all the testing for my heart gave me a clean bill of health. That was when I realized that these crushing chest pains that I was experiencing were heart burn. So now I make sure to pay more attention to possible food triggers that may be causing this pain.

My mother had always suffered from severe heart burn. She had all the classic symptoms and it seemed like no medications were working. She was having difficulty sleeping because the acid from her stomach wouldn't stay down. The doctor suggested that she may need surgery (fundoplication) to repair the esophagus flap to help keep the acid down.

Around the same time that I was on the transformational path to taking control of my life my mother went for hemocode testing that tested her for foods to which she may be allergic or sensitive. She discovered that there were a lot of foods with which she was having problems. After she started following a new strict diet of almost no grains (which were the grains related to gluten) and many other foods she was amazed to find out she had no more heart burn problem and even went off some of the pills that she had been taking for as long as I could remember. This shows that what we eat can change our lives for the better or make it a pill popping adventure that is no fun and can lead to other complication or possible side effects.

Symptoms of Heart Burn

Burning sensation in chest and upper abdomen

Burning feeling in throat

Feeling of food stuck in throat, esophagus or even in the upper chest

Chest pain (remember that this pain may be mistaken for heart attack. If you have chest pain and have never been told you have heart burn then you should get it checked out immediately, especially if you have any other symptoms of heart attack)

Irritable Bowel Syndrome (IBS)

Irritable Bowel Syndrome (IBS) is a condition in which the body behaves in an abnormal way without showing any underlining disease. It affects the GI tract and bowel movements. There is no clear cause of IBS. Theories include combinations of gut-brain axis problems, gut motility disorders, pain sensitivity, infections including small intestinal bacterial overgrowth, neurotransmitters, genetic factors, and food sensitivity. Onset may be triggered by an intestinal infection or stressful life event.

Finally, after years and years of ongoing suffering I was diagnosed as having IBS. I was grateful that I finally knew what was causing my problems, but remember IBS is a syndrome not a disease so there is no clear or specific treatment. Nothing changed, even after eliminating many of the foods that were suggested to me. Keep in mind that there was no talk of gluten or celiac disease in the public or among most doctors at that time. So, I remember when I had to go back to the doctor after being told I had IBS to express that I was not getting better (It wasn't good). This is when I had one doctor tell me it was all psychological. He said I should look at the way I was handling stress or take a pill. After that I never wanted to see any doctors for anything. I just could not face another doctor undermining me.

No one should have to feel the way I did, so keep pushing them until you are satisfied with the results. And most of all until you feel truly better. Just like fibromyalgia many people are wrongfully diagnosed with IBS when it is really celiac disease or gluten intolerance. And remember IBS is not a disease so it does not have a clear diagnosis and treatment. It is merely a statement that the bowel is irritated without determining any underlying cause. The proposed remedies are best guess to alleviate the irritation.

Symptoms of (IBS)

Pain and discomfort in the abdomen

Diarrhea

Constipation

Bloating

As you can see, the symptoms of IBS are the same as some symptoms of celiac disease

Kidney Disease

Kidney Disease causes the kidneys to not filter the blood properly to remove extra water and waste and pass it in the urine. If you have kidney disease you have probably already been told that changing your diet could help, and like many other conditions I have discussed, removing gluten may be helpful for some.

Symptoms of Kidney Disease

Loss of appetite

Reduced urination

Fatigue and weakness

Shortness of breath

Nausea

Pain in chest

Swelling of hands and feet

Lactose Intolerance

Lactose intolerance is a condition in which people have symptoms due to a decreased ability to digest lactose, a sugar found in dairy products, due to lower levels of lactase (the enzyme which breaks down lactose) production in the small intestine. Those affected vary in the amount of lactose they can tolerate before symptoms develop.

Lactose malabsorption means the body does not have sufficient lactase capacity to digest the amount of lactose ingested. Hypolactasia (lactase deficiency) is distinguished from alactasia (total lack of lactase), a rare congenital defect.

Lactose intolerance is not an allergy, because it does not cause an immune response, but rather a sensitivity to dairy caused by lactase deficiency. Milk allergy, occurring in only 4% of the population, is a separate condition, with distinct symptoms that occur when the presence of milk proteins trigger an immune reaction.

Symptoms of Lactose Intolerance

Diarrhea

Bloating

Gas, cramping

Gastroesophageal reflux (Throwing Up)

Liver Disease (NAFLD)

NAFLD stand for Non-Alcoholic Fatty Liver Disease and it occurs when fat builds up in the liver. The main function of the liver is to help in digestive processing and distribution of the nutrients from food. Risk factors include diabetes, obesity, a diet high in fructose and older age. Once again changing diet should bring improvement.

Symptoms of NAFLD

Loss of appetite

Yellowish appearance of the eyes and skin (Jaundice)

Swelling in legs, feet and ankles

Nausea

Vomiting

Fatigue

Abdominal pain and swelling on the right side

Lupus

Lupus is an autoimmune disease. Lupus occurs when the immune system starts to attack healthy tissue, causing inflammation and damage to joints, skin, kidney, blood, heart, brain, and blood vessels. Lupus and celiac disease share similar biomarkers, so you might be able to benefit from eating a gluten free diet. Just like celiac disease Lupus is very hard to diagnose.

Symptoms of Lupus

Muscle pain

Joint swelling and pain

Chest pain

Hair loss

Purple or pale toes and fingers

Fever

Red rash

Sun sensitivity

Swollen glands

Headaches

Confusion

Dizzy spells

Migraines

Migraines are a severe form of headache. They cause intense pulsing or throbbing pain on one or both sides of the head and sometimes disturb vision. The link between migraine and celiac disease could be because of the malabsorption of nutrients and inflammation. There is usually a reduction in occurrences and severity when on a gluten free diet. Other foods may also be triggers.

Symptoms of Migraines

Nausea

Vomiting

Sensitivity to light

Sensitivity to sound

Multiple Sclerosis (MS)

Multiple Sclerosis is an autoimmune disease that affects the central nervous system. This autoimmune disease causes the body to attack a fatty white substance, called myelin, that protects and insulates the nerves in the spinal cord and brain.

Symptom of MS

Fatigue

Numbness

Problems with bowels

Dizziness

Electric shock sensations

Pain in parts of the body

Speech impediments

Tingling or prickling feelings

Myasthenia Gravis

Myasthenia Gravis is an autoimmune disease that affects the skeletal muscles, causing painless weakness. It is caused when antibodies made by the immune system interrupt the nerve impulses to the muscles.

Symptoms of Myasthenia Graves

Muscle weakness in legs, arms, feet, fingers and neck

Problems talking

Difficulty swallowing or chewing

Shortness of breath

Facial expressions may change

Double or blurred vision

Drooping eyelids

Fatigue

Osteoporosis

Osteoporosis is a condition in which there is bone loss or loss of density, thus increasing the risk of fracture, cracking and breaking. Sometime there are no symptoms until a bone is broken. Once again, because of malnourishment from celiac disease or gluten intolerance there is an increased inability to have optimal bone density.

Symptoms of Osteoporosis

Stooped posture

Height loss

Pain in the bones

Loss of bone density

Psoriasis

Psoriasis is an autoimmune disease that affects skin cells. Psoriasis happens when the skin cells become overactive, causing them to pile up on the surface before they even have a chance to reach maturity. This causes inflammation, scaling and red patches on the skin. It usually affects the knees, elbows, scalp, legs, feet, hands, face and lower back. Like all autoimmune diseases the chances of having a link to another autoimmune disease is higher. As well some people with psoriasis have had great success eating a gluten free diet.

Systems of Psoriasis

Inflammation and swelling

Scaling of skin

Pain

Itching of the skin

Skin feels hot

Raynaud's Phenomenon

Raynaud's Phenomenon is a condition that affects the blood vessels in the extremities causing discolouration of the skin and numbness or tingling (pins and needles). This usually only affects the toes, fingers and ears but some people experience it in the legs and arms as well. There will be a colour change in the affected areas, usually they turn white or blue and then slowly turn red when the circulation returns and blood starts flowing back into the affected areas. This usually happens because of temperature changes from hot to cold but stress can cause it to happen as well.

My experience with Raynaud's was crazy and very extreme. It affected me so often that I had to use gloves when taking things out of the fridge and freezer. I started to find that even going from cold to hot would cause a flare up. I also wasn't lucky enough to have it only affect my finger and toes, it was also almost always in my feet and hands and, on rare occasions, it would spread to my legs and arms as well. This rare occurrence usually only happened when I would go swimming in a cold pool or wake boarding on the river. I would have to be the last one out on the board because we would immediately have to head back to shore after my turn. I always kept a house coat, towels, wool socks and a blanket to wrap up in on the boat. This was so that I could get the blood flowing again before we arrived back on shore because if I didn't, I wasn't able to walk. Have you ever tried to walk when your legs have fallen asleep? It just doesn't work. The second-best thing to finding out that my problem was gluten was that my Raynaud's disappeared completely as I removed gluten from my diet. I couldn't believe I could get rid of the gloves and not have to suffer from this problem any more. But I did find that if I accidentally had gluten it came back quickly. I hope this helps you because even if you're not celiac and you have this problem you could try to eliminate gluten – it is worth a try.

Symptoms of Raynaud's Phenomenon

Discoloration (paleness)

Sensation of cold and/or numbness

Sarcoidosis

Sarcoidosis is a disease involving abnormal collections of inflammatory cells that form lumps, known as granulomas, in the body's organs. It is said by some to be related to autoimmune diseases but the exact mechanism of this relationship is unknown. It usually affects the lungs and lymph nodes but has been known to affect other organs as well. The possible link to celiac disease is that celiac is an autoimmune disease. As well that bad word - Inflammation - pops up again and gluten and other foods can play a big part in causing inflammation in many locations in the body.

Symptoms of Sarcoidosis

Enlarged lymph nodes

Chest pain

Shortness of breath and difficulty breathing

Dry cough

Headaches

Dry eyes

Dry skin and rash

Vaginal dryness

Thyroid problem

Join and muscle pain

Numbness and tingling in legs and arms

Schizophrenia

Schizophrenia is a mental disorder that affects a person's

interactions with other people, how a person thinks, how they feel and causes a failure to recognize what is real from what is not. There is a good chance that following a strict Gluten free diet can help with the disorder.

Symptoms of Schizophrenia

Hallucination

Dysfunctional thinking and feeling

Delusions

Trouble with speech

Scleroderma

Scleroderma is a group of different rare Autoimmune Diseases that cause abnormal growth to the connective tissues causing hardening or thickening of the skin. It may only affect the skin, but could also affect the digestive tract, internal organs and blood vessels.

Symptoms of Scleroderma

Stiff, painful joints

Hardening or thickening of skin

Raynaud's phenomenon (small blood vessels are constricted)

Calcinosis (calcium deposits)

Esophageal (the esophagus not functioning proper)

Sepsis

Sepsis is caused by an overwhelming immune reaction to an infection. Sepsis usually occurs when the body has an infection or a medical condition. There may be a moderate risk of getting Sepsis if Celiac Disease developed as an adult. But that would only be when the immune system wasn't working right.

Symptoms of Sepsis

Fever

Chills

Rash on skin

Rapid breathing

Increased heart rate

Low platelet count

Sjogren's Syndrome

Sjogren's Syndrome is an Autoimmune Disease that causes the body to attack the glands that produce moisture, such as tears and saliva. Some people have benefited from being on a gluten free diet.

Symptoms of Sjogren's Syndrome

Dry mouth

Dry eyes

Dry skin and rash

Vaginal dryness

Thyroid problem

Joint and muscle pain

Numbness and tingling in legs and arms

Thrombocytopenia (Low Platelets)

Thrombocytopenia is a disease in which the platelet count in the blood is low. Platelets are the part of the blood which performs the clotting function. Like red blood cells they are produced by the bone marrow. Platelets have a life of only about 10 days so they are continually being produced and replaced.

Symptoms of Thrombocytopenia

Easy or excessive bruising

Superficial bleeding into the skin, appears as a rash of pinpoint- sized, reddish-purple spots (petechiae), usually on the lower legs

Prolonged bleeding from cuts

Bleeding from gums or nose

Blood in urine or stools

Unusually heavy menstrual flows

Fatigue

Enlarged spleen

Jaundice

Thyroid Disease

Thyroid Disease has two common types that could have an association with celiac disease. The two types are Graves' disease and Hashimoto's disease - one is an overactive thyroid (Graves') and one an underactive thyroid (Hashimoto's). Both are autoimmune diseases and have a strong connection with celiac disease. However, the connection is not often looked at.

Symptoms for Graves' Disease

Weight loss

Rapid pulse

Restlessness

Diarrhea

Insomnia

Irritability and nervousness

Feeling hot

Symptoms of Hashimoto's Disease

Weight gain

Slowed pulse

Confusion

Mental slowness

Thick and coarse hair

Feeling cold

Red puffy eyes

Heavy menstrual periods

Fatigue

Tuberculosis (TB)

Tuberculosis is an infectious disease that is spread from person to person though the air. TB mostly affects the lungs but also could affect other areas of the body. TB is more common in people who are malnourished and therefore people with untreated celiac disease are at a higher risk for getting TB if they come in contact with the virus.

Symptoms for TB

Prolonged coughing which causes chest pain

Coughing up blood

Fever

Weight loss

Fatigue

Night sweats and chills

Turner Syndrome

Turner Syndrome is a condition that affects only females. It occurs when there is a partly or completely missing X chromosome. People with Turner's syndrome may also have celiac disease.

Symptoms of Turner Syndrome

Short stature

Non-functioning ovaries

Swelling of hands and feet

Heart and blood pressure problems

Kidney problems

Osteoporosis

Short neck with a webbed appearance

Soft nails that turn up

Ulcerative Colitis

Ulcerative Colitis is an autoimmune disease in which your immune system sends out white blood cells to attack your inner intestinal lining, causing inflammation or ulcers in your colon. There is a strong link associated with celiac disease and often your doctor will suggest you follow a gluten free diet and low residue diet. *This is another autoimmune disease I have and am working hard to keep myself in remission.*

Symptoms of Ulcerative Colitis

Abdominal pain

Abdominal cramping

Diarrhea

Rectal bleeding

Weight loss

Fatigue

Urgency to defecate

Vitiligo

Vitiligo is an autoimmune disease in which the body's immune system may destroy the melanocytes (a mature melanin forming cell) in the skin, causing white patches to appear on the skin. This could affect any part of the body. There may be a connection with celiac disease and following a gluten free diet has been helpful for some.

Symptoms of Vitiligo

White patches anywhere, but mostly on the mouth, eyes, genitals and rectum.

Williams Syndrome

Williams Syndrome is a genetic disorder from birth that affects many parts of the body. There will be learning difficulties and very distinct facial features. There will be an overly friendly personality with high levels of anxiety and empathy. People with William Syndrome sometimes also have a greater chance of having celiac disease. So, if William Syndrome is suspected and there are digestive problems get tested.

Symptoms of Williams Syndrome

Heart defects

Failure to gain weight appropriately in infancy

Low muscle tone

Widely spaced teeth

Long philtrum (vertical indentation in middle of upper lip Between nasal septum and tubercule of upper lip)

Flattened nasal bridge

[92]

Highly verbal relative to their IQ

Overly sociable

Individuals hyper focus on the eyes of others in social engagements

CHAPTER 9

YOUR FUTURE LOOKS BRIGHTER

I hope that after reading the previous eight chapters you now have answers to some of the previously unanswered questions you may have had. I'm hoping that if you are thinking you have celiac disease, wheat allergy, gluten intolerance, or you already know you have one of the above, that you have taken some steps to regain control of your life.

My whole intention in writing this book is to give you more knowledge than I had before I started this journey - because I spent way too many years suffering. It would be great if you could eliminate unnecessary trips to the doctor's office or stop being wrongfully diagnosed, and even better, stop being told that it's all in your head. If you start taking some of the steps in this book it could mean a whole new wonderful chapter in your life. Imagine how much better you will feel, how wonderful you will look, and best of all, you would finally be on the road to doing what's right for your body.

Now, in saying that, I do want to make sure to help the people who are still not receiving answers or results about the causes of the bloating and unnecessary pain. I know this is something that does affect many of us - myself included. Even if you have taken gluten out of your diet it could take a year or longer for your body to heal. It most likely will be longer if you have been suffering with celiac disease or gluten intolerance for a long time and didn't know it. Some of us still continue to have ongoing symptoms, even after having passed the time frame for normal healing and having been completely free of gluten for that whole time. There is still hope. You just have to examine everything you eat or use much more closely.

When I first started on this journey, I was always accidentally contaminating myself. It is not that I wasn't trying, and I still have the occasional mishap. In chapter 6 I mentioned things that you might not know contain gluten. Or you might just forget. Things like the new toothpaste you bought because it was on sale (it's not like it's a food item). It could be that someone bought you some new face cream or makeup as a gift, and once again you just can't get it in your head that it may contain gluten. There were many items that I didn't know had gluten in them, and even when I had a list that I carried around with me I wouldn't remember to look at the list. If you are like me and found out before 2010 that you had a gluten problem, then you may not have had a list, and if you did it seemed to be much smaller. Any lists you come across today are way more informative and include many more products. I can't express enough to be very mindful of what you are eating, taking as vitamins or supplements, or applying to your skin. So read labels, ask questions or call the company.

When you are still experiencing problems after you have done your best to eliminate gluten there could still be something wrong - referred to as Non-Responsive Celiac Disease (NRCD). This is when the body is not responding to a gluten free diet and there are still symptoms. As well test results will still show evidence of damage to the intestinal villa. There could be reasons why this is happening to you. You may have another digestive disease or disorder. You may still be contaminating yourself as I explained at the beginning of this chapter and in chapter 6. Or it could be a problem with another food. You could be like me, and many others, who have a huge list of foods to which you are allergic or intolerant to. If you are still continuing to have problems that are unexplained your doctor may recommend a steroid as treatment to help heal the inflammation in the intestines.

Casein (a component of dairy products) is one of the hardest things for people with celiac disease to digest. You should consider getting tested for food intolerances rather then going though a process of elimination diet again. You may have found it hard to do, as I did, but if you want to do the process of elimination diet again you should make sure you only introduce

[95]

one item at a time and wait for a period of days to make sure your body is not responding. You should make certain dairy, grains and sugars are the last to be reintroduced.

For me the feeling is different when I've eaten something that has contaminated me with gluten compared to something to which I'm intolerant. I will know within 15 minutes of having consumed gluten, the pain I feel is like no other pain. I feel that I'm going to have to take a trip to the hospital. The funny thing is that the pain seems much more intense now, than when I didn't know I had celiac disease. One doctor told me that it is because you now know what normal is supposed to feel like. She also mentioned to me that the better you eat and take care of your body the more you will become aware of every little thing going on inside your body. This will help you identify possible triggers. I used to think that my body had built up a tolerance to gluten but I now know that it was me not listening to my body and putting up with the pain.

If you listen to your body it will tell you the difference between having something with gluten and having foods to which you are intolerant. This is what I am observing in my body now. When I have food, my body is intolerant to I experience bloating, inflammation, diarrhea or constipation, and sometimes cramping. I sometimes make the occasional choice to eat foods that cause me these problems. The times I choose are normally on my birthday and special occasions and I will have a gluten-free cake that contains sugar, so I suffer because of the choice I made. Almost all processed gluten-free products contain sugar. I have finally come across a bread that is sugar free O'Doughs original sandwich buns (gluten free, vegan, no added sugar, no trans fats, and non gmo). This bread is amazing and causes me no problems. Giving up sugar was harder then when I gave up gluten but this bread made it a little easier.

If you read my story in chapter 7 under constipation you would know that this could also be a major problem that you are experiencing and you may not even be aware of it. Let me just recap - sometimes when you are severely bloated, cramping, feeling nausea, decreased appetite as well as an inability to pass gas and you think you are experiencing diarrhea it could be a partially obstructed bowel (impacted stool). Partial Bowel obstructions occur when a mass of hard dry stool is unable to pass through the colon or rectum and you could still be passing a watery loose stool a couple of times a day.

When your intestinal villi have been damaged, they may absorb more water from the stool because of the inability to absorb the nutrients, which could help to contribute to constipation or a partially impacted stool.

There is also the fact that when you are following a strict gluten free diet that you are not getting enough fibre in your diet because lots of the processed gluten free products you are using as replacements don't contain the high fibre contents you need to make sure constipation doesn't occurs.

This was the case for me, the doctor suggested I go on a high fiber diet. I added foods like flax seed, oats, nuts, quinoa, chickpeas, hemp seeds and berries. Eliminate gassy foods like brussel sprouts, broccoli, cabbage, cauliflower, onions, pears, soft drinks, all dairy and most beans. Eliminate fried foods, oils and margarine, and that will help heal the inflammation in the intestines. I also added more fermented foods to help with good gut health. As well as an evening laxative like smooth move tea with Senna. I increased foods like prunes, kiwifruit, figs, apples, and citrus fruits. Make certain they don't cause you gas. It was also recommended that I add psyllium to my diet - this is a sure way for you to get your daily fibre intake and it's foolproof. The doctor felt that I should follow this diet for about 3 months because I needed to retrain my bowels to function properly. After following this high fiber diet, I found that some of the foods that I was once sensitive to no longer bothered me. This was thanks to the healing of my irritated bowel and the constipation was now gone.

When it came to having to take an evening laxative, I had to go with something mild and natural like Senna which is herbal tea that works by gently stimulating your intestines and helping in the natural elimination process. Also, fennel, peppermint and ginger can help as well. When I was taking things like polyethylene glycol, bisacodyl and docusate I found I was experiencing side effects like headaches and bloody stool. These different laxatives do things like draw water to soften the stool and stimulate the bowel muscles. If you are planning on trying something that's not natural, like I suggested, just make sure it claims to be certified as totally gluten free. And also drink lots of water.

This is another suggestion you may want to consider. My husband and I have tried to give up all meat and fish products, eggs, refined flours and foods with added sugars, added fats and oils, and dairy. This is called a Whole Foods Plant Based Diet (occasionally we still have a little sugar or oil). We made this positive life choice after reading the China study by Colin Campbell and watching related documentaries such as forks over knives. My husband has seen positive changes in his health and weight. I was also able to see that it benefited my healing process as well.

I have listed the foods that this diet consists of below if you would like to give it a try. But I do recommend you check out the web sites I have listed below if you are really interested.

Fruits: apple, banana, blueberry, prune, fig, pear, strawberry, raspberry, avocado, orange, apricot, blackcurrant, blackberry, lemon, lime and many more awesome fruits. To choose from a more detailed list refer to chapter 6 under the list of fruits you can eat on a gluten free diet.

Vegetables: asparagus, bok choy, broccoli, kale, cabbage, peppers, celery, zucchini, turnip, mushroom, spinach, carrots, cauliflower, collard greens, and leek. Once again there are many more to choose from, refer to chapter 6.

Starchy vegetables & tubers: potato (all kinds), whole corn, peas, quinoa and taro.

Legumes: every kind of beans and lentils.

Whole grains: oats, brown rice, wild rice, red or black rice, buckwheat, millet, and many more. But keep in mind that if you have to eliminate gluten stay clear of the grains that contain it also listed in chapter 6.

Seeds and nuts: cashew, walnut, hazelnut, almond, pumpkin seed, sesame seed, flax seed and chia seed.

Beverages: water, unsweetened plant smoothies, decaffeinated coffee and tea

Spices: all are good to consume

This may be a life style you want to consider for optimal healing of the body. But for starters you may just want to eliminate the foods that are causing your body discomfort. It is now time for you to make up your mind whether you want to travel this path. Get tested and you will be one step closer to having freedom from inflammation in the body and all your tummy troubles.

I would love to support you as much as possible through the process because I know it's always easier if you have someone that has gone though it to talk to. You can contact me on Facebook at http://www.facebook.com/TheGlutengal/ or you can join me on http://www.instagram.com/theglutengal.info or http://www.twitter.com/theglutengal. I'm sure if you come and join me there will be someone out there that has gone though the same things you are going though, if I haven't. If you are interested in learning more about the Plant Based Diet I would suggest visiting https://www.forksoverknives.com/what-to-eat/. There are also many support groups for the Gluten Free community as well as the Whole Foods Plant Based Community listed in the resources at the back of this book. Support in numbers is much better than trying to do it on your own. My wishes are that you will find strength, happiness and peace in your new journey.

Thank-You, Thank-You, Thank-You.

Chapter 10

My Little Miracle

For those of you who have made it this far in the book this is the story I told you I would share about everything my husband and I went through trying to have a baby, who turned out to be our wonderful son Richie. It took a while before I became pregnant, but it was not something we considered a problem. When I finally became pregnant, we were very excited. I had done everything I could, eating the right nutrients and taking all the prenatal multivitamins with folic acid before I started trying to get pregnant. I was still eating my enemy, gluten, which I didn't know was my enemy at the time. I was doing everything possible to ensure the perfect pregnancy. So, you can understand why I was so devastated and confused when I had a miscarriage at about 10 weeks. If you have ever experienced a miscarriage you know the pain of losing your baby.

Once I was pregnant again, I did everything to ensure that I was living a healthy lifestyle, just like my first pregnancy. I was having no problems at all and was thoroughly enjoying it. I loved having my baby boy in my tummy. I talked and sang to him every day and it was like he was responding to my every word.

I was now 29 weeks and all my appointments with the doctors had been great. It was Wednesday, Oct, 7 1998 and I was at work. I began to feel sick to my stomach and was having trouble with my vision. I decided to go home, but because of the type of person that I am I didn't want to make a big deal out of something that was probably nothing. I went home and slept for about 16 hours, waking the next morning when I had to go back to work. That Thursday at work I was feeling back to normal not realizing that I was in the calm before the storm.

It was now Friday and my husband and I went to my sister-in-law Debbie's family cottage. We were there to help with a project to repair the boat house, as well as to enjoy a little R&R on the beautiful lake. We were only there about 3 hours when I started to feel sick, with a tummy ache and diarrhea again. I went and laid down with the hope that I would shake this crummy feeling. I do have a very fond memory of my time laying there. My niece Madison, only 5 at this time, was very concerned and empathetic about my condition. It was a precious moment for me, as she talked my ear off and ran her little fingers though my long hair. Her caring little heart, kept my mind in a very warm happy place that helped me forget about the discomfort that I was feeling.

A couple of hours later I was feeling a little better and joined all my loving family. We all sat down to enjoy an Indonesian dish called bami goreng that a close family friend, Marcel, had prepared for us. It was delicious, and of course, contained gluten. About an hour after dinner I started to feel sick once again, and as much as I wanted to be able to enjoy the camp fire I had to excuse myself and go to bed early. That was when things became worse. I had severe diarrhea and started vomiting. I had crushing chest and diaphragm pain, trouble breathing and felt extremely unwell. I thought maybe I had food poisoning. I didn't let anyone know how bad things were until I started to see blood in the toilet from when I was vomiting, urinating and having bowel movements. At this point I knew I was in serious trouble because I was only 29 weeks pregnant. That was when I asked my husband to please take me to the hospital.

We were 40 min away from the hospital but we knew it would be faster to drive than to wait for an ambulance. It was the longest most painful journey that I had ever experienced in my life. I felt like I was dying and I didn't think my baby was going to make it because it was much too early in my pregnancy. It was late at night, really dark and raining extremely hard. I remember this one moment a beautiful deer coming down a hill and sliding out onto the road, it looked just like a scene from the movie Bambi when Bambi slid across the ice. Thank God my husband drives for a living and managed to avoid hitting the deer. When we arrived at the hospital, they took me right into emergency. Luckily the doctor on call had an idea of what might be happening to me. He was at home and relayed the instruction to the nurse over the phone.

My blood pressure was 240 over 150 and four days ago, at the doctors my blood pressure was 100 over 50 which is normal for me. I was bleeding internally, felt like my chest was in a vice and was drifting in and out of consciousness. I remember one moment very clearly. I was feeling very calm, and it was surreal (like a dream) as I watched the events unfold around me. The nurses were rushing around frantically, fiddling with the tubes and equipment that were hooked up to me. I also remember seeing my husband in the corner of this little room with a look of horror on his face.

My husband recalls watching me turn blue on the table as he listened to the nurses yelling that my blood pressure was not going down. He remembers when the doctor came running in and instantly started following the intravenous tube and realized the hose was kinked. As soon as the doctor unkinked the hose it was only seconds before I turned pink again. This is when my husband said he felt like he could breath once again. I don't remember anything after that but thank God there was an amazing doctor on call. They explained to my husband that they had concluded I had H.E.L.L.P syndrome, which is very hard to diagnose, especially 20 years ago (1998). I hadn't heard of it and I'm sure most other people hadn't heard of it either.

H.E.L.L.P syndrome stands for Hemolysis, Elevated Liver enzymes, and Low Platelet count. H.E.L.L.P is thought to be a complication to preeclampsia but also occurs for unknown reasons. They explained to my husband that once they could stabilize my blood pressure, they would perform an emergency Cesarean section to deliver the baby in order to keep me alive. The doctor told my husband If the baby remains in your wife, her body is going to continue to shut down and that she may not survive.

They performed an emergency C-section and my son was delivered weighing 2 lb 6 oz. He was very sick, couldn't breath on his own and his skin was still transparent. My son had so many things wrong that he had to fight with all his might to survive. An aeromedical unit was sent Because this was only a level #2 hospital . One doctor and two nurses stabilized my son Richie for transport to a level #3 hospital that could care for a premature baby of his small size. When I woke up, they brought my little boy to me so I could touch his tiny hand – At the time I couldn't even see him because my eyesight hadn't yet returned.

The next week was very long as I fought for my recovery with blood transfusions and many tests to see what kind of damage had been done to my organs, brain and eyes from the H.E.L.L.P syndrome, which also caused me to have a mini-stroke, called a Transient Ischemic Attack (TIA). Six days later my blood pressure was down and I was finally stable enough to be released.

This is a day I will never forget and can call upon whenever I need to feel happy and grateful. What I felt when I stepped out of the hospital on that glorious beautiful October day was pure blissfulness. I tipped my head back and felt the amazing warmth of the sun shining down on my face. The smell of fresh air filled my nose and made me thankful that I was breathing. Now that my eyesight had returned, they were lit up by the intense, brilliant and bright fall colours that cascaded all around me. This was a magical moment and I remember the feeling of pure love and gratitude for being alive in my heart and soul. I had never ever experienced anything of this magnitude in my whole life. Thank you thank you, thank you to all the people who cared for me and kept me alive, and for all the caring and generous people who donate the life saving gift of their blood.

When I arrived at the hospital where my son was being treated, I felt even more joyous. My mother told me later that it was the most heartfelt thing she had ever seen. The first time my little boy heard my soft voice he tried to open his tiny eyes to see where I was and his little hand opened to reach for mine. As I am writing this, I have tears running down my cheeks as I recall the feeling of love and joy that filled my heart. This was an amazing day and it will always be imprinted in my memory.

My son still had an uphill battle. He was on a respirator to help him breath, his skin was transparent and you could see all his tiny veins. He also had a feeding tube and many, many wires hooked up all over his little body. It was a long 2 months in the hospital, with many ups and downs, before he came home. He is now 20 years old and didn't suffer any complications that affected his health. He will always be my little miracle and I'm so very grateful to have my son in my life. My son is an amazing gift that has changed my perspective on life time and time again.

Thank You Richie.

I am also thankful for our health care system and for every single nurse and doctor who cared for him.

It took about one year for me to recover from the TIA and internal bleeding, and for my organs that had started to shut down to recover, all of which was brought on by the H.E.L.L.P syndrome. It was very challenging and difficult to overcome all the things I experienced and had to relearn because of the mini stroke. But because of my little miracle I found the strength and determination to persevere and be a better person than I was before. And become the most loving caring mother I could be so I could provide him with all that he deserved.

There has been some research suggesting a possible association with autoimmune dysfunction and H.E.L.L.P syndrome. I hope there will be more research done in the future, so that no one else will ever have to go though what I consider the hardest, most excruciating event of my life. But also, one of the very best. I would like you to consider the possibility of whether or not you have celiac disease or gluten intolerance before you get pregnant, because it may save your life, or your baby's, or both, considering that both H.E.L.L.P syndrome and a baby being born prematurely can be life threatening to both mother and child.

I hope you have enjoyed this story about Richie, my precious little miracle.

Chapter 11

Gluten Free Recipes

I thought I would include some recipes that you might like to try. My husband, who is a chef, and I created these and use them occasionally.

Smoothies

Green Apple Smoothie

2 cups unsweetened apple juice
1 cup kale
1 cup spinach
1 avocado peeled and pitted
1 apple
2 tbs (30g or 1 oz) pea protein isolate
1 tsp cinnamon

Combine all ingredients in a blender and mix well.

Blueberry Almond Smoothie

2 cups unsweetened almond milk
1 banana peeled
2 cups frozen blueberries
1 cup kale

1 cup spinach

1 tbs ground flax seed

½ tsp cinnamon

¼ tsp ground or fresh ginger

Combine all ingredients in a blender and mix well.

Banana Smoothie

2 ½ cups unsweetened almond milk

½ cup almonds, blanched

2 bananas

1 tsp cinnamon

1 tsp vanilla

1 tbs flax seed

Combine all ingredients in a blender and mix well.

Mixed Berry Smoothie

2 cups unsweetened almond milk

2 cups frozen mixed berries

1 cup spinach

1 banana peeled

5 pitted dates

2 tsp cinnamon

½ tsp ground fennel seed

2 tsp (30g or 1 oz) of pea protein isolate

Combine all ingredients in a blender and mix well. With every one of these smoothies the ingredients can be changed to suit your needs. The type of protein used can also be changed. These are all approximations because there are so many brands.

Examples:

30 g (1 oz) of each of the following contain:

Whey protein: 115 calories, 20g protein, 5g carbohydrates, 1.5g fat

If you are on a Plant Based Diet or vegan diet

Pea Isolate: 120 calories, 24g protein, 1.2g carbohydrates, 1.8g fat

Soy protein: 110 calories, 25g protein, 1.5g carbohydrates, .5g fat

Flaxseed, ground: 160 calories, 5g protein, 8g carbohydrates, 10g fat

   Remember this will vary by brand. Remember to read the ingredients to ensure there is no wheat (gluten).

Recipes

Hot Flaxseed Porridge

¼ cup ground flaxseed

¼ cup boiling water

¼ cup chopped dates

¼ cup almonds chopped or whole

¼ cup chopped walnuts

 1 tsp cinnamon

1 tbs shredded coconut

1 tbs raw honey or maple syrup

½ cup unsweetened almond milk

1. Add boiling water to flaxseed and whisk until it is all blended smoothly.
2. Add remaining ingredients and mix well.
3. Then pour almond milk on top.

Macaroni Bean Salad

2 cups uncooked corn, rice, or quinoa (for gluten free) or whole wheat macaroni noodles

1 540 ml (19 oz) can kidney beans drained and rinsed well

1 540 ml (19 oz) can black beans drained and rinsed well

2 celery stalks, chopped

½ green pepper, chopped

½ red pepper, chopped

½ yellow pepper, chopped

1 small red onion, chopped

Sauce:

½ cup distilled vinegar

1 tbs tomato paste

1 tsp of gluten free soy sauce

½ tsp salt

1 tsp pepper

1 tsp chili powder

1 garlic clove minced

2 tbs apple cider vinegar

1 tsp lime or lemon juice

1 tsp ground cumin

1. Cook noodles in pot of boiling water until tender, drain and cool.

2. In a large bowl combined cooked noodles, beans, chick peas, chopped onion, celery, green and red peppers.

3. In another bowl combined distilled vinegar, tomato paste, soy sauce, ground cumin, chili powder, garlic clove, apple cider vinegar and lemon or lime juice.

4. Pour sauce over noodles and bean mixture, mix well, refrigerate and serve cold.

Gluten-free Fritters

1 cup gluten free flour

1 ½ tsp baking soda

¼ tsp salt

½ tsp pepper

½ tsp rosemary

½ tsp thyme

½ tsp garlic powder

1 egg or egg replacement or 1 tbs flaxseed beaten into 3 tbs hot water

¾ cup unsweetened soy milk

1 ¼ cups chopped onions (1 large onion)

1 540 ml (19 oz) can chick peas (garbanzo beans) drained and rinsed

½ cup mashed potato

¼ cup shredded carrots

¼ cup chopped spinach

sunflower oil or vegetable stock for frying

1. Combine flour, baking soda, salt, and pepper, rosemary, thyme and garlic together.

2. Add soy milk, mashed potato and egg or egg replacement or flaxseed/water and beat until smooth.

3. Stir in chickpeas, shredded carrots, chopped onions and spinach.

4. In a non-stick frying pan heat oil or veg stock at medium heat.

5. Add a tablespoon of mixture and cook approximately 5 min. until golden brown.

Potato Salad

8 large potatoes, peeled

3 ripe avocados, peeled and pitted

2 small onions, chopped

5 dill pickles, chopped

2 celery stalks, chopped

1/3 each red, orange, yellow and green pepper, chopped

1 carrot, shredded

½ tsp pepper

½ tsp salt

1 tsp thyme

1 tsp fresh dill, chopped

4 tbs gluten free mustard

1. Place peeled and quartered potatoes into a large pot and boil for about 10 to 12 min.

2. Remove and cool immediately in cold water.

3. Cut into cubes.

4. Cream the avocados in a large bowl.

5. Add mustard, salt, pepper, thyme, chopped dill and blend.

6. Add shredded carrots, chopped onions, pickles, orange, red, yellow and green peppers, mix well.

7. Fold in potato cubes.

8. For best results refrigerate overnight or at least a couple of hours.

9. Serve cold.

Tomato Vegetable Soup

2 1600 g (48 oz) cans tomato juice

2 840 g (28 oz) cans diced tomatoes

1 165 g (5.5 oz) can tomato paste

1 ½ l water or vegetable stock

10 carrots, peeled and chopped

2 green pepper, chopped

1 red pepper, chopped

1 yellow pepper, chopped

3 stalks celery, chopped

3 onions, chopped

1 cup broccoli

2 parsnips, chopped

1 cup spinach, chopped

1 cup kale, chopped

½ turnip, chopped

2 cabbage, chopped

4 green onions, chopped

½ cup lentils

1 garlic clove or 1½ tsp of powder

3 tsp salt

1 tsp onion powder

1 tsp basil

1 tsp marjoram

1 tsp oregano

2 tsp pepper

2 bay leaves

2 tbs maple syrup, if plant based
If not plant based 4 tbs sugar

2 tbs vegetable oil or vegetable stock to sauté
vegetables

2 tbs gluten free beef stock

4 tbs gluten free chicken stock

1. In a large pot add oil or vegetable stock. Using medium heat sauté in this order: onions, garlic clove, celery and then peppers.

2. When the vegetables are soft add tomato juice, diced tomatoes, tomato paste, water or vegetable stock and all spices.

3. If plant based add maple syrup (sugar, beef and chicken stock if you are not following a plant based diet).

4. Now add all remaining vegetables and lentils, bring to a boil. Cook until carrots, lentils and turnip are tender. Cook in a large pot on stove or a slow cooker.

Black Bean and Lentil Soup

2 l. water (to cook lentils)

2 l. vegetable stock

1 840 g (28 oz) can diced tomatoes

2 cups dry whole lentils

¼ cup vegetable oil or vegetable stock for plant based

1 onion, chopped

2 large carrots, peeled and chopped

2 stalks celery, chopped

1 cup green peas

1 cup kale, chopped

1 cup spinach, chopped

1 cup black beans, cooked

½ cup whole lentils

2 cloves garlic, minced

1 tsp oregano

1 bay leaf

1 tsp salt

1 tsp pepper

1 tsp basil

2 tbs red wine or apple cider vinegar

3 tbs chicken stock (if not plant based)

1. In pot bring water and dry whole lentils to a boil. Cook for 20 minutes.
2. Put cooked lentils in a blender or mix until creamy, set aside.
3. In a large pot add oil or vegetable stock. Sauté garlic cloves, onion, celery and carrot on medium heat.
4. Add vegetable stock, creamed lentil mixture, canned tomatoes, spices and chicken stock, bring to a boil.
5. Add whole lentils, black beans, peas, kale, spinach, and red wine vinegar. Cook until carrots and lentils are cooked then serve hot.

Vegetable Stir Fry

1 cup yellow onions, chopped

1 cup red onions, chopped

1 cup celery, chopped

1 cup carrots, chopped

1 cup cauliflower pieces

1 cup broccoli pieces

1 cup each red, yellow, orange, and green pepper

1 cup snow peas

1 cup chopped zucchini

4 tbs of oil or vegetable stock

1 cup water or vegetable stock

1 tsp salt

1 tsp pepper

1 tsp marjoram

1 tsp thyme

3 tbs gluten free chicken base or for vegan use 2 all vegetable bouillon chicken cubes, or none for plant based

1. Add 3 tbs of oil or vegetable stock to a wok and heat on medium heat.

2. Add red and yellow onions to wok and sauté for 3 min.

3. Add carrots and celery and sauté for 10 min.

4. Add peppers and sauté for 3 min.

5. Add cauliflower, water or vegetable stock, and spices.

6. Simmer on low for 4 min.

7. Add zucchini, snow peas and broccoli. Simmer on low for 8 min. or until everything is cooked. Serve over a bed of rice or noodles

Support Groups National and International

Canadian and American

Autoimmune Disease Support Group	www.inspire.c
Autoimmune Disease Support Group Facebook	http://facebook.com@AutoimmuneDiseaseSupportGroup
Academy of Nutrition Dietetics	www.eatright.org
American Celiac Disease Alliance	http://americanceliac.org
Asthma and Allergy Foundation of America	www.aafa.org
Beyond Celiac	www.beyondceliac.org
Canadian Celiac Association	www.celiac.ca
Celiac Disease Foundation	www.celiac.org
Celiac Support Association	www.csaceliacs.info
Celiac Support Group Facebook	http://facebook@CeliacSupportgroup

Gluten Free Celiac Disease Support Group	http://facebook @GlutenFreeCeliacDiseaseSupportGroup
Gluten Intolerance Group	www.gluten.org
National Digestive Diseases Information Clearinghouse (this is my favourite website)	http://digestive.niddk.nih.gov
National Foundation for Celiac Awareness	www.celiaccentral.org
R.O.C.K (Raising Our Celiac Kids)	www.celiac.com

International

Argentina	http://www.celiaco.orgiar/
Australia	http://www.coeliac.org.au/
Austria	http://www.zoeliakie.or.at
Belgium	http://www.sbc.asbl.be/
Brazil	http://www.acelbra.org.br/eng

	lish/index.php
Croatia	http://www.cel ijakjja.hr/
Cyprus	annatsoia@cyt anet.comcy
Czech Republic	http://celiac.cz
Denmark	http://www.co eliaki.dk/
Europe	http://www.ao ecs.org/
Finland	http://www.kel iakialiitto.fi/
France	http://wwwafdi ag.fr/index.php
Germany	http://www.dz g-online.dc
Greece	http://www.co eliac.gr/
Hungary	http://www.co eliac.hu/tiki-index.php
India	http://celiacsoc ietyrajasthan.c om
Ireland	http://www.co elic.ie
Israel	http://www.cel iac.org.il/

Italy	http://wwwceliachia.it/home/homepage.aspx
Luxembourg	http://www.alg.lu/
Malta	http://www.coeliacassoeiationmalta.org/
Netherlands	http://www.glutenvrijinl/
Norway	http://www.ncf.no/
Pakistan	http://celiac.com.pk/index.php
Poland	http://wwwceliakia.pl/
Portugal	http://wwwceliacos.org.pt/
Russia	http://www.celiac.spb.ru
Saudi Arabia	http://www.saudi-celiac.com/main/
Slovakia	http://wwwceliakia.sk/uvoc/
Slovenia	http://drustvo-

	celiakija.si/
Spain	http://www.celiacscatalalunya.org//
Sweden	http://celiaki.se/
Switzerland	http://www.zoeliakie.ch/
Tunisia	http://atmc.org.tn/atmc@topnet.tn
Turkey	http://www.colyakie.ch/
Ukraine	http://www.celiac-ukraine.com/
United Arab Emirates	http://wwwglutenfreeuae.com/
United Kingdom	http://www.coeliac.co.uk
Uruguay	http://www.acelu.org

Alphanumeric Index

Cancer
24,25,64,69,75

Candida
64,70,71

Canker sores
47,49,52,61

Casein Allergy
64,71

Cognitive Impairment
64,72

Constipation
18,21,23,47,49,51,52,53,71,78,96

Crohn's Disease
24,25,56,64,72

Depression
7,21,31,48,49,53,54,66

Dermatitis Herpetiformis
48,49,53

Diabetes Types
60,61,64,73,74,81

Diarrhea
4,18,21,23,34,48,49,52,62,66,71,73,78,81,89,91,96,101
Down Syndrome
64,74,75

Dyspepsia (Acid Reflux)
21,62,64,75,77

Eczema
64,75,76

Epilepsy
61,64,76

Fatty stool
48,56

Fibromyalgia
64,76,77,78

Flatulence or gas
23,48,49,50,51,52,56,70,75,81

Headaches
18,48,49,52,54,57,66,71,82,86,98

Heart Burn
64,77,78

Infertility
48,49,57

Irritable Bowel Syndrome
9,64,78

Itchy, Watery Eyes
47

Kidney disease
64,80

Lactose Intolerance
56,64,71,80,81

Liver disease
56,64,81

Lupus
64,81,82

Migraines
64,72

Miscarriage
48,49,58

Menopause
48,50,58,59

Menstrual periods
 48,50,58,59,61,66,89,90

Multiple Sclerosis
64,83

Myasthenia
64,83

Nausea
21,23,48,49,52,56,60,66,73,75,80,81,82,96

Numbness, tingling hands & feet
50,60,74,86,88

Osteoporosis
52,65,66,84,91

Psoriasis
65,84

Puberty
48,61

Raynaud's Phenomenon
50,60,65,85,86,87

Sarcoidosis
65,86

Schizophrenia
65,86,87

Scleroderma
65,87
Seizures
8,48,50,60,76

Sepsis
64,87,88

Sjogren's Syndrome
65,88

Slowed Growth
48,62,75

Thrombocytopenia Low Platelets
8,65,88,89

Thyroid, pancreatic & Hashimoto disease
65,68,88,89,90

Tuberculosis
65,90

Turner syndrome
65,91

Ulcerative Colitis
48,50,61,91,92

Ulcers and sores
48,50,61,91,92

Vitiligo
65,92

Weight loss & gain
7,21,23,30,48,51,54,62,66,69,73,74,89,90,91,92

Williams syndrome
65,92,93

Yeast Infections
70,71

About the Author

Cindy Martin was born and raised in Toronto Canada. She loves to share and interact with others on Facebook at http://www.facebook.com/TheGlutengal/ as well as http://www.instagram.com/theglutengal.info or on http://www.twitter.com/theglutengal.

Cindy has battled with digestive disorders all her life, which has led her to way too many visits to the doctor office with multiple tests having been done. Cindy has researched this topic for over 10 yrs with the hopes of being able to make sense of what she had been experiencing all her life, only to find out that this stuff called gluten was a huge contributor to her disorders.

Cindy has transformed her life from being full of pain and depression by learning to heal her body and has been able to allow happiness and joy into her soul. Which has helped her to thrive in a gluten free world. Cindy has also started to write her next book which will help you in the healing of your body carrying you onto the next steps of healing your mind.